MEASURING HEALTH STATUS

MEASURING HEALTH STATUS

Sonja M Hunt, James McEwen and Stephen P McKenna

CROOM HELM
London • Sydney • Dover, New Hampshire

© 1986 Sonja M. Hunt, James McEwen and Stephen P. McKenna
Croom Helm Ltd, Provident House, Burrell Row,
Beckenham, Kent BR3 1AT

Croom Helm Australia Pty Ltd, Suite 4, 6th Floor,
64-76 Kippax Street, Surry Hills, NSW 2010, Australia

British Library Cataloguing in Publication Data

Hunt, Sonja M.
    Measuring health status.
    1. Medical care − Evaluation
    I. Title II. McEwen, J.   III. McKenna, Stephen P.
    362.1   RA399.A1
    ISBN 0-7099-3584-6

Croom Helm, 51 Washington Street, Dover,
New Hampshire 03820, USA

Library of Congress Cataloging in Publication Data

Hunt, Sonja M.
    Measuring health status.

    Includes bibliographies.
    1. Health status indicators. 2. Health surveys.
3. Nottingham health profile. I. McEwen, James.
II. McKenna, Stephen P. III. Title. (DNLM:
1. Health surveys. WA 900.1 H943M)
RA408.5.H86   1986   362.1′072   85-29950
ISBN 0-7099-3584-6

Printed and bound in Great Britain
by Billing & Sons Limited, Worcester.

CONTENTS

Acknowledgements
Introduction

1. HEALTH TRENDS AND HEALTH SERVICES   1

   The Changing Patterns of Health and
      Illness...............................   2
   Lay and Professional Attitudes to Health   4
   The Orientation of the Health Services
      and their Problems of Adaptation......   7
   The New Public Health Challenge:
      Inequalities in Health...............   11
         Health Promotion Opportunity and
            Realism...........................   13
   References...............................   17

2. PLANNING FOR HEALTH AND RESOURCE
   ALLOCATION

   The Theoretical Background..............   20
   Planning and Information in a Health
      Service...............................   24
   Health Care - What are the Objectives?..   32
   References...............................   35

3. MEASURING HEALTH STATUS   37

   Mortality Rates.........................   39
   Morbidity Measures......................   40
   Refined Indices.........................   41
   Disability Indices......................   42
   Symptom and Function Indices............   44
   The Search for a Global Index...........   52
   Choice of a Health Indicator...........   54
   References...............................   56

Contents

4.   SELF REPORT AND SUBJECTIVE HEALTH STATUS   61

Evaluating Health Status................   63
Perceived Health and Health Outcome.....   68
References..............................   70

5.   DEVELOPING AN INDICATOR OF PERCEIVED
    HEALTH   75

Selecting Items for Inclusion in a
Perceived Health Measure................   76
Selection of Method of Scaling..........   77
Developing Indices from Scaling Methods   80
The Development of the Nottingham Health
    Profile...............................   85
    Weighting the Statements..............   87
    Validity and Reliability.............   95
Consulters and Non-consulters of General
    Practitioners.........................   98
Studies of 'Fit' Populations............ 102
The Development of Part II of the
Nottingham Health Profile............... 107
    Patients Recovering from Fractures.... 109
    Reliability Testing................... 113
Conclusions............................. 117
References.............................. 119

6.   MEASURING PERCEIVED HEALTH IN THE
    COMMUNITY............................... 124

Establishing Norms for the Nottingham
Health Profile.......................... 124
    Norms for a General Practice.......... 125
    Adapting Norms for Comparison......... 129
    Norms for an Employed Population...... 130
    Extending and Updating Norms.......... 132
Population Studies Employing the
Nottingham Health Profile as an
Established Research Tool.............. 134
    Intra-Urban Variations in Health...... 134
    The Perceived Health of Unemployed and
    Employed Workers..................... 139
Problems associated with Community
    Studies............................... 148
    Sample Size and Sampling.............. 149
    Non-Response.......................... 150
    Accuracy.............................. 153
Distribution of scores on the NHP....... 154
Conclusions............................. 160
References.............................. 160

Contents

7.   HEALTH INDICATORS IN CLINICAL CARE   163

     Deciding on Treatment...................   164
     Differing Expectations of Care..........   168
     Reviewing 'Normality': The Case of
        Pregnancy............................   174
     A New Treatment.........................   181
     Monitoring Progress in Problematic
        Situations...........................   195
     The Potential Value of the Nottingham
        Health Profile.......................   196
     References..............................   200

8.   CROSS-CULTURAL ISSUES IN HEALTH
     INDICATORS   203

     Mortality Rates.........................   204
     Morbidity...............................   206
     Socio-medical Indicators................   207
     Questionnaires and Interviews...........   210
        Conceptual and Linguistic Issues.....   211
        Translation..........................   211
     An Arabic Version of the NHP............   213
     A Spanish Version of the Sickness Impact
        Profile..............................   217
     A Spanish Version of the NHP............   218
     A North American Version of the NHP.....   219
     Conclusions.............................   221
     References..............................   222

9.   THE USE AND ABUSE OF HEALTH INDICATORS   225

     Health Indicators in Priority Setting...   226
     Ethical Considerations in the Use of
        Health Measures......................   227
     The Concept of Positive Health..........   230
     The Nottingham Health Profile:
        Retrospect and Prospect..............   231
     Conclusions.............................   238
     References..............................   238

     APPENDIX   241

     The Nottingham Health Profile...........   241
     User's Manual...........................   246

ACKNOWLEDGEMENTS

The authors are grateful to the Economic and Social Science Research Council for their financial support of the developmental work on the Nottingham Health Profile. (Grant No 6157/1). We owe a debt to Carlos Martini and Ian McDowell who carried out the initial research and to Jan Williams and Evelyn Papp who worked so tirelessly and imaginatively to keep the projects running smoothly.

Maurice Backett has our deepest respect and affection for his suggestions and constant support during our time in the Department of Community Health at Nottingham.

We also thank Jocelyn Greer-Spencer for her speedy typing, Leslie Alexander for her constructive criticisms and Katherine Melia for her patience and diligence in the preparation of the final manuscript.

To the several members of the medical profession who made facilities available to us and co-operated willingly in our research we are also grateful.

All those many members of the public who patiently gave of their time, volunteered their opinions and made all this possible are gratefully acknowledged.

We are grateful for permission to reprint figures and tables from 'Costs and Benefits of the Heart Transplant Programmes at Harefield and Papworth Hospitals' by M. Buxton et al, published by HMSO, 'Crown Copyright Reserved (C), 1985.

INTRODUCTION

A common characteristic of health services throughout the world, is that, regardless of financing or type of provision, health and medical services have operated without any systematic or continuous evaluation of their impact on the health status of the patients they treat, the communities in which they are set, or the nation as a whole. Moreover, the services which are provided often seem to have evolved out of chance occurrences, become hallowed by time and perpetuated by inertia. A relationship between health services and the health status of clients is assumed rather than known.

The realisation that universal, easily accessible medical care does not automatically abolish the inequalities of health and the soaring cost of maintaining health systems, has led lately to the recognition that clear objectives need to be set for health, medical and social services. These objectives should be based upon information of a high quality rather than upon tradition and hunch. Built in to the data collection and goal setting there is a need for a continuous monitoring and feedback system, such that assessment of the link between objectives, processes and outcomes can be made.

There is now general agreement that setting objectives to reduce ill health and promote good health is largely a matter of defining needs and evaluating the extent to which needs are met or could be met by the health system. The evaluation of services, whether at community or clinical level is attracting increasing interest - in theory, if not yet in practice - although the means and methods by which such evaluation could or should be carried out remain controversial.

Problems of defining need and from whose

perspective, together with the known association between availability and demand, have made the search for 'objective' criteria of need a fruitless enterprise. The belated recognition that it is 'subjective' need which plays a major role in utilisation of services has led to a general acceptance that perceived benefit should play a crucial role in assessing the efficacy and efficiency of services and that perceived need could be of great value in planning health care and resource allocation.

Routinely kept statistics concerned with the health of a population such as mortality rates, death and discharge rates and hospital admissions figures are becoming increasingly unhelpful in an era of longevity and where chronic rather than acute illness dominates the medical scene. Moreover, in industrialised countries some of these routine statistics are now so low (for example, maternal mortality rates) as to be quite inappropriate as a basis for decision making, although they are still important in the monitoring of specific areas of clinical care.

These issues, together with greater pressure from lay persons, the wish to have information about those individuals who do not seek medical attention and the costs of certain medical techniques and health strategies of unproven worth, have given rise to calls for the production of new methods of health status assessment.

It is against this background that the development of the Nottingham Health Profile took place. The Profile was the culmination of an attempt to utilise self-reported distress to measure the 'subjective health status' or 'perceived health' of individuals, groups and communities. The rationale behind the development of the Profile, the methods used in its validation and reliability testing and the uses to which it is being put are described here as an illustration of one response to the need for new measures of health. General points about the methodology of instrument design, particularly in relation to choice of items, validation, weighting of scores and standardisation are also demonstrated.

Besides providing an overview of the current state of the art in health indicators research the book is set in the current conceptual and practical framework of health services provision and medical intervention and discusses the advantages and limitations of using measures like the Nottingham

Health Profile in population surveys, clinical care and the evaluation of health services.

Chapter 1 deals with the current orientation of medical and health care and the problems associated with the adaptation of traditional modes of service delivery to contemporary trends in patterns of ill health and changes in population structure. The need for a more psychosocial emphasis in defining health is discussed together with the issue of who is regarded as having responsibility for health.

Chapter 2 takes up the issues of planning and allocation in health services and the basis on which decisions are made, both internationally and locally. The establishment of a common health policy by the World Health Organisation with its need for a sound information system is described. The promise of Community Medicine and its failure to live up to that promise leads to a consideration of the requirements necessary for efficient, equitable and sensitive strategies for health care. The chapter comments on the perpetuation of social inequalities in health status and their implications for health promotion and the distribution of resources in a primary care setting.

In chapter 3 issues of defining health and illness lead to a description of the several ways in which attempts have been made to measure and assess health status. Starting with mortality statistics and routine morbidity assessment the chapter goes on to describe and evaluate various types of health indicators, including disability indices, symptom and function rating scales, quality of life measures and various health and sickness profiles, including methods of assessing mental health. The interest of health economists in a single, global index of health is noted and the chapter concludes by setting out some criteria by which a health indicator might be selected for research purposes.

The various philosophical and methodological problems associated with using subjective health measures, based on self report are described in chapter 4. The traditional distinctions between 'objective' and 'subjective', 'mental' and 'physical', 'internal' and 'external' are set in the context of the domination of a particular view of science and the expansion of the medical profession. Studies comparing lay and professional opinions of some medical outcomes suggest discrepancies and various trends have led to demands that lay perspectives be given a greater emphasis in the provision of services and the evaluation of

outcomes. The role of perceived need in utilisation
of medical and health care and the predictive value
of self-assessed health status are discussed.

In chapter 5 the rationale and methodology
behind the the Nottingham Health Profile are used to
illustrate issues in the development of a health
indicator including techniques of scaling;
collection and choice of items, methods of weighting
items to reflect severity and gives details of
various studies used to assess validity and
reliability of the Nottingham Health Profile
including the health of the elderly, consulters and
non-consulters of a general practitioner, fracture
victims and the perceived health of 'fit' workers
such as firemen and mine rescue workers. The
development of norms for comparison is described in
chapter 6 which concludes by detailing some of the
practical uses to which the Profile has been put,
including assessment of the need for health care in
the inner city, social inequalities in health and
comparisons of employed and unemployed people.

Specific clinical applications of the Profile
make up chapter 7 which considers some of the
problems associated with the use of such an
indicator in the clinical setting. Research design,
ethics, the interpretation of results and the
appropriateness and value of subjective measures are
discussed. Studies mentioned here include the heart
transplantation programme of Harefield and Papworth,
use of the NHP with cancer patients and an
investigation of quality of life during pregnancy.
Since the completion of the NHP there have been many
requests to use it from other countries, including
the USA, Taiwan, Holland, Spain, Sweden and Egypt.
The adaptation of a subjective health measure for
use in another culture, or even in sub-cultures of
the same society poses serious problems of semantic
and conceptual equivalence. Chapter 8 deals with
these problems in the context of cross-cultural
comparisons of health status and ethnomedicine.
Differences in the definition, classification,
experience and diagnosis of disease are discussed.
The translation of questionnaires and interviews
requires, in addition, strict adherence to a set of
criteria for achieving linguistic and semantic
relevance and attempts to translate the NHP into
Arabic, Spanish and 'American' are described as well
as the successful production of a 'chicano' version
of the Sickness Impact Profile.

The book concludes with a consideration of some
of the issues arising out of the use of health

indicators. These include the dangers of the 'medicalisation' of social problems, the focus on negative aspects of health experience, ethical aspects of the administration of health questionnaires and the use of subjective measures in priority setting. The advantages and limitations of the Nottingham Health Profile are summarised and the future prospects for its use are surveyed.

The Appendix contains the NHP itself together with a user's manual which gives summary details of the development of the questionnaire, mean scores of various groups, age and sex norms and a description of a computer programme for converting responses into weighted scores.

Chapter 1.

HEALTH TRENDS AND HEALTH SERVICES

In every country, the link between the changing pattern of health and the provision of health care is a matter of regular debate, but frequently, the evidence to sustain the argument is limited or absent. Definitions of health are regarded as inadequate, the relationship between health and quality of life is uncertain and the value and adequacy of health care is debated by individuals, health professionals, pressure groups, economists and government. The mass media extol rapid scientific medical advances. Television programmes on health and health care gain high viewing figures. The stark picture of poverty, malnutrition and early death in the developing countries is reflected in paler form in social inequalities in health in western society. The paradox between the dramatic improvements resulting from medical and surgical technology and the inability to reduce the burden of chronic disease, particularly in an increasingly elderly population, is apparent. At the same time there is a new scepticism and anxiety relating to health care and how it will cope with new demands and rising expectations. All these changes have implications both for those who provide care and for the recipients.

This chapter will not attempt to produce a comprehensive or chronological account of the changes that have taken place and are still occurring, but rather, will pick out a few examples of change where uncertainties exist, where explanations are still incomplete or lacking and where more sensitive measures of health might be useful in determining need and assessing the outcome of care - both at individual and community levels. Concern with cost containment, the emphasis on management efficiency, public desire for good quality care and the increasing interest in involvement by patients and the general public in all aspects of health care have contributed to this quest for better measures of need and outcome.

THE CHANGING PATTERNS OF HEALTH AND ILLNESS

Until the nineteenth century, patterns of health and illness were determined largely by the influence of infectious diseases against the background of the physical environment and the state of nutrition both of which were in turn closely related to social class and poverty. McKeown (1980) and other writers have drawn attention to the fact that many of the advances in health have been related more to socio-economic, environmental and educational changes than to medical intervention. During the nineteenth and early part of the twentieth centuries, the public health movement achieved marked improvements in the health of the community through action aimed at the societal level. Those involved in public health accompanied by the social reformers showed that the individual could make only a small contribution to health and that social action was required to eradicate dangerous and harmful working environments, cover open sewers and provide pure drinking water. Developing skills in preventive medicine, bacteriology, engineering and education were used by the social reformers to reduce the spread of communicable disease, produce better housing, healthier and safer working and living conditions and improved nutrition. These developments were followed by health education, child health services, and the development of effective vaccines and immunisation programmes more directly involving the individual.

Following the public health movement with its emphasis on prevention of disease, there were marked advances in medical treatment. Initially, this was in the field of infectious disease with the development of chemotherapy. The antibiotics provide one of the best examples of a group of drugs that can ensure complete cure. Following treatment of many serious infections, the patient returns to a normal life - a life which without the antibiotic might not have existed or where the effects of the infection might, untreated, have resulted in some permanent disability. Side effects are relatively rare or minor for most antibiotics. The effect of these magic bullets in acute disease and the consequent extension of life expectancy has resulted in a relatively increased burden of chronic multi-causal degenerative diseases where inevitably cure has been more elusive. Although increasing technical developments relating to all kinds of disease have enabled practitioners in the health services, in hospital and community, to intervene more effectively in many of the chronic diseases, it is often more accurate to regard the treatment as leading to amelioration of the impact of the disease or as halting or slowing its progress, rather than effecting a permanent cure.

Such advances have led in turn to changes in the population structure. Worldwide there is an overall increase in population and in western societies, the main impact is from the relative increase in dependent groups, particularly the elderly. Projected populations in the United Kingdom (Office of Population Census and Surveys, 1984) show a continuing increase in the number of persons aged 75 years and over, with this becoming particularly rapid in the second decade of the next century. The number of persons of younger pensionable age is projected to decline a little by the year 2001 but to increase sharply in the first two decades of the next century. Thus there is an increasing number of very frail persons who may be either physically or mentally handicapped or both.

Although as indicated, dramatic cures are unlikely because of the inherent nature of chronic diseases, there is the possibility of dramatic reduction in the effects of such conditions.

Two surgical procedures introduced in recent years show how rewarding new techniques can be, and how patients, formerly inevitably committed to severe disability or death, can now hope for a much improved life. Hip replacement operations have ensured enormous reduction in pain and increased mobility in many older patients enabling them to remain independent and lead a fuller and more normal life. Renal transplantation and the associated advances in chemotherapy have prevented premature deaths and ensured satisfying social and effective working lives in many younger patients. The problems of the availability of kidneys for transplant and the facilities for dialysis either before, or as an alternative to transplant, still remain and are consequent largely upon the allocation of resources to health care.

However, in many chronic conditions an individual may have to cope with a permanent

3

handicap or require continuing medication to ensure survival. In conditions such as diabetes or renal dialysis, the patient, often supported by family members, assumes a major role in managing the problem on a day to day basis by the monitoring and management of diet and by adjusting way of life.

With certain progressive diseases such as the cancers, there may be several options in treatment. These may range from simple palliative treatment which will reduce the unpleasant symptoms of the disease, but is unlikely to improve the prognosis, to extensive surgery or repeated courses of chemotherapy which may offer increased years of survival but will be associated with greater risk at the time of treatment and possible serious side-effects, disfigurement or handicap.

All these changes have implications for patients, their families, professionals and those who plan health services. Patients and their families will wish to know the options - the risks and the benefits, professionals will have to be able to impart this information to their patients and those providing the service will be required to assess priorities and be more sensitive to the patients' perspective and their assessment of need.

With technological advances, whole new areas are drawn into the medical domain. Conception, its prevention or encouragement had little to do with health professionals until the discovery of the contraceptive pill, the advent of the IUD, legal termination of pregnancy and in-vitro fertilisation. The ethical, moral and technical dilemmas arising from such advances are debated by government, professionals, church and pressure groups, frequently with little understanding of the issues involved, the needs of clients, the outcomes of alternative techniques or the impact on clients of these medical techniques.

LAY AND PROFESSIONAL ATTITUDES TO HEALTH

The limitations of the old negative definition of health 'as the absence of disease' have long been recognised, but some health professionals, either, when looking after individuals, or when planning health services for a community, still seem to be unaware of the wider implications. Herzlich (1973) has argued for a psycho-social orientation which is centred upon the articulation of the person and the socio-cultural system. She notes that:

Anthropologists and historians of medicine are in general agreement that causal conceptions of illness - whether popular notions or medical theories - range between two extremes. On the one hand, illness is endogenous to man, and the individual carries it in embryo; the idea of resistance to disease, heredity and pre-disposition are the key concepts. On the other hand, illness is thought of as exogenous: man is naturally healthy and illness is due to the action of an evil will, a demon or sorceror, noxious element, emanations from the earth or microbes, for example.

Herzlich in interviews with a sample of the French public found three concepts of health. The first 'health in a vacuum' was a state of <u>being</u> involving absence of illness; the second was the idea of a 'reserve of health'- a state of <u>having</u> the positive aspects of strength and robustness; the third was a state of <u>doing</u> involving physical well being and social relationships and was seen as 'equilibrium of health'.

The first concept corresponds to some extent to the medical view, the second includes the ideas of fitness going beyond biological health, while the third raises expectations about quality of life. Do the public now expect health care to provide for all aspects of health needs, and how do the professionals define need for care? The failure to recognise the different approaches to defining need together with uncertainty about the relationship between need and health care planning remains as a source of conflict and confusion between patients and professionals.

Magi and Allander (1981) suggested that statements of need should be classified on the basis of who makes them. They have proposed a primary classification of <u>self assessed need</u> (an individual's assessment of his own situation) and <u>other assessed need</u> (the assessor and the assessed are not the same person). They consider that total congruence on the individual level between self and other assessed need is not possible because of the unique and introspective character of self assessed need. They further suggest that, in medical practice, this incongruence tends to be increased due to the difference between the patient and the doctor with regard to general social background, specific knowledge and experience of ill health, technical competence and ability to control utilisation of medical care. This is illustrated by the term 'perceived illness' as the lay concept of ill health while the medical concept is described as 'observed disease'. In summary, the most important determinants of assessment of for what and when one should seek medical attention are assumed to be the assessor's perception and valuation of health status and the expectation of the probable outcome of medical care use. Thus these two 'needs' are relevant both to the provision of individual health care and to the planning of health services for a community.

In attempting to describe health no single approach is likely to be comprehensive. Professional descriptions based on physical or biological departures from normal and professional estimates of the effect that such departures have on an individual must be seen against the individual's perspective on feeling and functioning. Generally, doctors have been less interested in debating definitions of health and have been more concerned to measure the 'hard', 'objective' data, such as the biochemistry of patients, the range of movement in an injured or arthritic limb, the improvement in the radiograph or the time taken for an injury to heal. Similarly, the patients may be equally uninterested in the debates on risk factors or attributions of cause and are most alarmed by subjective feelings and reductions in activities associated with everyday life.

Both 'objective' and 'subjective' perspectives can be equally valid in describing states of health, but the inability to quantify 'subjective' health meant that patients' perceptions were often dismissed and reliance was placed on 'objective' measures. These important issues are developed more fully in chapters 3 and 4. The construction of valid and reliable measures of perceived health now provides an opportunity to redress the imbalance. Researchers, administrators, patients and doctors may all have different perspectives on need and health, but the differences have not always been recognised by the others. Nor have they been taken account of in planning health care and services.

THE ORIENTATION OF HEALTH SERVICES AND THEIR PROBLEMS OF ADAPTATION

The early years of the nineteenth century saw the development of general practice and professional education for those involved in health care. This culminated in our present institutions and divisions of health and medical personnel. Health care became available to all. Prior to that professional care was mainly the prerogative of the wealthy. In rural areas, self care, at times supported by some local wise person with experience in traditional remedies or midwifery, was frequently all that was available. As both treatment and preventive techniques expanded, it was recognised that different methods and skills were required for the provision of preventive services to a community and for individual care of a sick person. At the same time, it was appreciated that the mass approach required in the prevention or control of disease had different administrative, legal and, at times, ethical considerations and consequently public health developed as a separate discipline. The provision of formal preventive and curative services did not, however, prevent much debate as to the responsibility of the individual for the avoidance of ill health. Currently, this separation still exists, although there is a tendency in many countries to try to bring together the preventive and curative services.

There are still major environmental, social policy and planning issues relevant to pollution, employment, nutrition, housing, town planning and industrial policies which require corporate action to improve health. While it is accepted that because there are behavioural aspects to ill health such as cigarette smoking and excess use of alcohol, some of the initiatives lie with the individual, involving personal decisions to change behaviour, there are at the same time political and economic considerations which encourage both smoking and drinking (Taylor, 1984). It is also to be recognised (Cameron and Jones, 1985) that 'drugs of solace' are not only necessary to relieve individuals of great burden of pain and suffering, but that society in its present form could not function without them.

Virtually all the significant advances in treatment can be achieved only with considerable expenditure on equipment, drugs, highly trained staff and supporting services. Research programmes and service expansion have frequently been dictated by the power and influence of senior doctors or by tradition and have not always been related directly to need. Consequently priorities have rarely been assessed. It is necessary for the optimum deployment of resources in social policy and in the planning of health care that there be some means of estimating levels of health and illness in a community and the distribution of ill health within different populations. Only then will it be possible to describe problems and priorities and test alternative solutions or types of care in an informed manner.

The public generally expect that the full benefits of medical science should be available when required. The problems of assessing priorities, rationing care and resolving the unequal distribution of services are difficult to understand -particularly when such services are vital for their survival or comfort. Virtually all technological advances produce a paradox. On the one hand, the increasing complexity and bureaucracy of the health services which accompany sophisticated medical technology means that more decisions are taken centrally by a few highly skilled people with greater responsibility being given to professionals and administrators. Patients may be seen by many people in different departments in a large hospital and this may create the impression of a cold, remote, uncaring scientific medicine. On the other hand, the emphasis on consumerism, self care and increased patient involvement can signify a greater responsibility for the patient and indeed may be seen as a response to the less desirable aspects of modern medical provision.

Consumerism and self care have had a significant influence on attitudes to health and health care (McEwen, Martini and Wilkins, 1983). The earlier movements sought to change the way that the country was governed and services provided, while later, the emphasis was based in 'grass roots' organisations and sought to improve the lot of the person or ordinary patient. Health was deemed to be too important to be left completely to professionals and politicians - the individual surely having the greatest commitment to his or her own health and body.

Probably the most important and by far the most widespread changes have been with the establishment of self help groups (Katz and Bender, 1976; Hatch and Kickbusch, 1983). Such groups emphasise the value of bonding together, the special expertise sufferers have gained through their experiences and the need for additional support, care or education in addition to that provided by the health services. As a result of having passed through crises and having coped with problems, members of self-help groups are able to help others with similar conditions and there is often a desire to turn what may have been a negative experience into something positive - both for themselves and for others.

Generally, such groups:

1. Provide support, comfort and therapy for members.
2. Provide practical care, courses, materials, education etc. not elsewhere available.
3. Act so as to exert pressure for change in national or local policies.

While self-help groups tend to be informal, spontaneous, limited in their objectives and sometimes short-lived, more formal aspects of consumerism exist. Within the health sevices in the United Kingdom, Community Health Councils have been established officially to provide the 'community voice' and have defined statutory responsibilities and funding. In some instances a localised and non-statutory group is established in health centres or general medical practices. These practice associations (Norell, 1980) have been set up to aid communication between patients, doctors, nurses and other staff, to participate in the running of the practice and to arrange educational sessions.

This move towards greater patient participation, the development of pressure groups and the changing attitudes towards professionals and bureaucracy has implications for those involved in social policy. Who has responsibility for prevention, health promotion and the provision of care? What is the contribution of the individual and what should be the contribution of government and authorities? With the current emphasis by government on 'cost cutting' and efficiency in the health services, there is often pressure for a greater part to be played by the individual in solving problems of self care, with family care and community care being seen as cheaper alternatives to institutional care. However, there is seldom an examination of the effectiveness of such alternatives. It is all too easy for authorities to seek to blame individuals and to transfer to individuals responsibility for collective failure. Illich (1975) considers that 'the level of public health corresponds to the degree to which the means and responsibility for coping with illness are distributed amongst the total population'.

Illich believes that 'medicine' and professions in general erode individual autonomy and are part of the hierarchy associated with social organisation and bureaucracy. He argues for a return to a 'free' economy with less access to health services, the freedom of people to choose any healer and the abolition of regulations governing the licensing of doctors. Navarro (1976) believes Illich places too much emphasis on <u>cure</u> instead of <u>care</u> and sees the power of bureaucracies as a symptom of industrial capitalism, not a cause:

> I would encourage you to think of social medicine and public health not only in terms of improving water and sewage systems, or even in terms of improving occupational medicine, but also and previously (as did the founders of social medicine) in terms of redistributing the economic and political power in our society from a few to the many. Indeed, Virchow, the founder of social medicine clearly saw the need to merge the medical task with the political and social faces. 'Medicine is a social science and politics is medicine on a large scale ....' In summary, I perceive the public health task as serving and supporting the public's demands not only for health resources, but also for control of these and all the resources they produce. But in order to undertake that task, it is necessary to realise that we cannot have a progressive health movement in the absence of a progressive political movement.

The philosophy behind the founding of the Welfare State in Britain was 'to divorce health care from personal finance or other factors irrelevant to health' (His Majesty's Stationery Office, 1944). Today, this philosophy still remains the basis of the service, although some changes have been made. Criticisms relating to inadequate funding, old fashioned hospital premises or staffing problems do exist but the benefits of such a system and its achievements should not be diminished by some of the deficiencies which are frequently fewer and less severe than those found in other countries where there are different systems of funding health care by insurance or where state provision is limited to the very poor. Whatever proportion of the gross national product is spent on health and irrespective of the system of funding, total funds are limited, and in some countries, decreasing. This is happening in the face of increasing demands for health care resources. In the United Kingdom, attempts have been made to remedy the problems in the National Health Service, by administrative restructuring - in 1974, 1982 and 1984. The current emphasis is on efficient management, but if this is to be more than political dogma, sound information is required to determine health needs and evaluate care - whether provided by the state system, private organisations or voluntary and charitable effort.

It is always tempting to believe that the latest re-organisation will remedy all the problems in the health services, but these dichotomies between state provision and self-help, so well portrayed by Illich and Navarro still exist, and indeed, existed in Victorian times. Is it possible that by making these more explicit through the current concern over inequalities in health and by seeking to integrate the twin aspects of health promotion - prevention and cure, that state provision and self-help could be made complementary instead of opposed? This could lead on to a more detailed examination of responsibility for care, how different groups make decisions and with what information, whether they be autonomous hospital consultants, isolated general practition-ers, governments or community health councils. Equally important is the responsibility for deciding on research priorities.

THE NEW PUBLIC HEALTH CHALLENGE: INEQUALITIES IN HEALTH

In virtually all countries there is growing concern about inequalities in health between socio-economic groups and between rich and poor countries. The health problems associated with social deprivation can be regarded as the major new public health challenge (Brotherston, 1975). The publication in the United Kingdom of the Black Report (Department of Health and Social Security,

1980) drew attention to the substantial and accumulating evidence that the differences in health status between higher and lower socio-economic groups as measured by morbidity and mortality indicators is becoming wider and this in spite of a National Health Service providing comprehensive, continuous and freely available health care.

Gradients of longevity and morbidity related to social class have been observed for centuries. Those in the lower socio-economic groups have had shorter life expectancy and higher death rates for almost all causes of deaths at least since the 12th century, when data on this topic were first collected and organised (Antonovsky, 1967). While it is true that mortality has declined somewhat for the poor, there has been an even greater decline in mortality for the better off, with the effect of widening the existing gap (Department of Health and Social Security, 1980).

National statistics, such as those collected by the Office of Population Censuses and Surveys and local studies in some of the deprived inner city areas have pointed to the many aspects of health and health care associated with social deprivation – higher rates of acute and chronic illnes, more and longer hospital admissions, greater use of general practitioner services, higher infant mortality, more accidents, more psychiatric disorders, more self reported sickness (Townsend, Simpson and Tibbs, 1984). These studies have shown an association of physical and material health problems with social indicators such as type of housing, overcrowding, social class, unemployment, the proportion of certain persons in the community – the elderly, the socially isolated, single parent families – and with poor primary care services, but further work is required to clarify the nature of the associations. In addition, studies should attempt to identify the characteristics of those exposed to deprivation who do and do not suffer from poorer health.

Early investigation by committed individuals, like Charles Booth in East London at the turn of the century, led to concern over slums and destitution in inner city areas. Today, this has continued through such schemes as Educational Priority Areas, Urban Aid Programmes, Partnership Schemes and Housing Action Area Programmes. These and other imaginative initiatives have done much to tackle specific problems, but it is often difficult to assess both the short and long term impact on health and less attention has been paid to the more dispersed aggregations of deprivation that exist in smaller towns and rural areas where the problems are qualitatively and quantitatively different. In addition to the concern over environmental issues in Victorian times, there was a parallel commitment to education and indirect behaviour change. Recently, a renewed importance has been attached to health education as a means of improving individual health, but there is concern that this may be merely a device by the authorities to displace responsibility on to the individual. It may also be seen as an attempt to 'medicalise' the problem by emphasising individual 'treatment'.

Health Promotion: Opportunity and Realism

Traditionally the aim of health education has been to encourage individuals to give up potentially damaging behaviour or to adopt an activity designed to promote health. Many health educators have been disappointed at their lack of success and it is all too easy to blame this on the ignorance, stupidity and irresponsibility of the public. Social scientists have criticised the 'victim blaming' approach - perhaps epitomised in traditional health education - which points to the aspects of individual behaviour associated with disease causation and prescribes a list of individual do's and don't's. As Pill and Stott (1982) point out:

> What is missing, however, both in the official documents and criticisms of them, is any discussion of how members of the general public may feel about the onus for illness being shifted on to the individual. The establishment of just what the concept of individual responsibility for health means to various groups in our society would seem to be a necessary first step in assessing how effective official policy on preventive health is likely to be and formulating appropriate strategies for behaviour change.

In their study of working-class mothers, Pill and Stott found that at least half held fatalistic views about illness causation and were prepared to accept the concept of blame only under very restricted circumstances involving direct risk taking. Three possible hypotheses are put forward to explain the failures of health education.

1. That a section of society is inevitably resistant to change and so fixed in their ways that personal changes are unlikely to be achieved.
2. That innovation in health education and prevention can still achieve better results with the 'resistant' sector of society.
3. That a large section of society is trapped in socio-economic circumstances which render the officially recommended choices of life-style either impractical or irrelevant, however much the individual may desire change.

More recently, the traditional emphasis on individual behaviour change has been associated with some of the less well thought out attempts at health promotion, with exhortations to individuals to change their ways in relation to exercise, relaxation or diet. This unbalanced emphasis on individual responsibility alone, although frequently popular with government, fails to take account of the acknowledged social, educational and epidemiological research that recognises the close relationship between individual behaviour and the social and physical environment -both of which affect health.

The Declaration of Alma-Ata (World Health Organisaton, 1978) speaks of developing programmes 'in the spirit of self-reliance and self-determination' and notes that these in turn must be based on the ability 'to participate individually and collectively in the planning and implementation of health care'. The foundation of this programme is to be primary health care with an emphasis on community participation and development, with water, agriculture, industry and education all being involved in addition to traditional primary medical care. The lessons being learned in the developing and under-resourced parts of the world, resulting in new methods of delivery of services, new categories of health worker and new approaches to health education, can encourage those in western countries to be more imaginative in tackling today's problems.

Primary care in the United Kingdom, albeit slightly narrower in concept and more medically orientated than in developing countries, has changed dramatically over the past thirty years, with new training programmes and multidisciplinary teams being seen as the focus for comprehensive and continuing care. From being essentially reactive to the medical problems presented by patients, it is now suggested that primary health care should assume responsibility for the health of the practice population and become pro-active through screening programmes, health education and greater participation by the practice population. The term anticipatory care (Royal College of General Practitioners, 1981) has been introduced combining prevention with care - care with an eye to the future. No other branch of medical practice exhibits such diversity in quality and scope of provision as is found in primary care. The primary health care approach lays great emphasis on health education, its development and integration with all health care and with community development in a concerted contribution to enhancement of quality of life. Kickbusch (1981) considers that 'we are witnessing at the moment a basic change in health education approaches' in the European Region of the World Health Organisation, and that this is reflected in four main conceptual re-orientations:

1. From health prescription to health promotion.
2. From individualistic behaviour modification to a systematic public health approach.
3. From medical orientations to recognition of lay competence.
4. From authoritarian health education to supportive health education.

Many people are not as optimistic as Kickbusch and consider that we are witnessing a few scattered attempts at change and that the change may not be as radical as the rhetoric implies.

However, such thinking led to the establishment in 1984 of a new programme in 'Health Promotion' in the WHO European Regional Office (World Health Organisation, 1984). The term health promotion has been adopted with enthusiasm by many in the United Kingdom, but frequently with inadequate thought and without consideration of a relevant theoretical framework. Some have regarded it as an opportunistic bandwagon (Williams, 1984). Some have emphasised the marketing of health, some have seen it as a superior, more comprehensive, variety of health education, while others have regarded it as a new revitalised successor to preventive medicine.

Such limited views are not only at variance with the changes mentioned by Kickbusch, but they fall short of the concept in the new WHO programme.

> At a general level, health promotion has come to represent a unifying concept for those who recognise the need for change in the ways and conditions of living, in order to promote health. Health promotion represents a mediating strategy between people and their environments, synthesising personal choice and social responsibility in health to create a healthier future.

(World Health Organisation, 1984)

It is to be hoped that such statements will be influential in the developing of health and health care and will not be regarded just as the result of irrelevant committee deliberations.

It is against this background of changing technology, a desire for participation, advances in prevention and alteration in provision of care that there have emerged demands for the tools to measure more effectively the need for health care at both the individual and community levels and to be able to evaluate the provision of such health care. Today, many issues resulting from the changing patterns of health and disease remain unresolved – why, for example, are the elderly and the mentally handicapped so badly catered for? Why is it that it has not been possible to decide on the most effective and most acceptable forms of care and what financial provision should be made available and for whom? Is it possible to predict the impact on health and quality of life of the proposed shift in care from hospital to community? What will be the overall impact of reduced resources?

The next chapter will examine the current state of information on health and illness and the ways in which decisions on service provision are made. Some of the advances mentioned are of obvious and proven worth, other approaches have become hallowed by long usage, while some of the newer changes are still untested. Those working in the health service are aware of the limited information available when discussions about priority programmes or major investments in buildings and equipment are being held. Is there a reasonably practical way to improve the quality of information available for planning the provision of care and for assisting individual patients in making decisions about their own care?

REFERENCES

Acheson, D. (1981) Primary Health Care in Inner London, Report of a study commissioned by the London Health Planning Consortium, LHPC, London

Antonovsky, A. (1967) 'Social Class, Life Expectancy and Overall Mortality,' Mil Mem F Quart, 45, 31-38

Brotherston, Sir J. (1975) 'Inequality: Is it inevitable?', The Galton Lecture, 1975 in C.O.Carter and J. Peel (eds.), Equalities and Inequalities in Health, Proceedings of the 12th Annual Symposium of the Eugenics Society, Academic Press, London, pp. 73-104

Cameron, D. and James, I.G. (1985) 'An Epidemiological and Sociological Analysis of the Use of Alcohol, Tobacco and other Drugs of Solace', Community Medicine, 7, 18-29

Department of Health and Social Security, (1980) Inequalities in Health: Report of a Research Working Group, HMSO, London

Hatch, S. and Kickbusch, I. (eds.), (1983) Self-help and Health in Europe, WHO, Copenhagen

Herzlich, C. (1973) Health and Illness. A Social Psychological Analysis, translated by D. Graham, European Monographs in Social Psychology, Academic Press, London

Her Majesty's Stationery Office (1944) A National Health Service, Coalition Government White Paper, Cmndd 6502, HMSO, London

Illich, I. (1975) Medical Nemesis: The Expropriation of Health, Calder and Boyars, London

Katz, A.H. and Bender, E.I. (1976) The Strength in Us Self-Help Groups in the Modern World, New Viewpoints, New York

Kickbusch, I. (1981) 'Involvement in Health: A Social Concept of Health Education', Int J Hlth Ed, 24, 3-15

Magi, M. and Allander, E. (1981) 'Towards a Theory of Perceived and Mentally Defined Need', Sociol Hlth and Ill, 3, 49-71

McEwen, J. Martini, C.M.J. and Wilkins, N. (1983) Participation in Health, Croom Helm, London

McKeown, T. (1980) The Role of Medicine: Dream, Mirage or Nemesis, Blackwell, Oxford

Navarro, V. (1976) Medicine Under Capitalism, Croom Helm, London

Norell, J.S. (1980) 'Patient Participation Groups', J Roy Soc Med, 73, 697-698

Office of Population Censuses and Surveys (1984) OPCS Monitor, PP2 84/1 Government Statistical Service, London

Pill, R. and Stott, N.C.H. (1982) 'Concepts of Illness Causation and Responsibility: Some Preliminary Data from a Sample of Working Class Mothers', Soc Sci Med, 16, 43-52

Royal College of General Practitioners (1981) Health and Prevention in Primary Care, Report for General Practice 18, RCGP, London

Taylor, P. (1984) Smoke Ring: The Politics of Tobacco, Bodley Head, London

Townsend, P. Simpson, D. and Tibbs N. (1984) Inequalities of Health in the City of Bristol, University of Bristol, Department of Social Administration, Bristol

Williams, G. (1984) 'Health Promotion - Caring Concern or Slick Salesmanship?' J Med Ethics, 10, 191-195

World Health Organisation, (1978) Report of the International Conference on Primary Health Care Declaration of Alma Ata, WHO/UNICEF I CPHC/ALA/78.

World Health Organisation, (1984) Health Promotion: A Discussion Document on the Concept and Principles, Regional Office for Europe, WHO, Copenhagen

Chapter 2.

PLANNING FOR HEALTH AND RESOURCE ALLOCATION

The differing attitudes that exist to the provision
of health care have been noted. The individual
practitioner, of whatever profession or training,
based either in hospital or community health
services, is concerned to be responsive to the
'demands' of the patient. Practitioners utilise
their clinical experience in deciding on the best
form of care for a particular patient. On the other
hand, those responsible for providing care to
populations or communities seek to determine the
overall 'needs' of the group, preferably quantified
in terms of morbidity and mortality and consider the
impact of alternative forms of provision. If
necessary, they can determine priorities related to
existing facilities and resources and examine the
possibilities for extending the overall programme of
care. This oversimplified view of the approaches to
the provision of care illustrates differential
requirements for information in making decisions,
yet in both cases, there has been a notable failure
to develop a systematic approach based on sound
information. Decisions, based on hunches, tradition
or personal power, have most frequently been the
norm and have rarely been subjected to rigorous
scrutiny. This chapter will be concerned mainly
with the planning of health care for groups,
communities or countries rather than estimating the
need for care at individual level.

In 'Health Crisis 2000' O'Neill (1983)
graphically describes the chaos in medical and
health care that exists in virtually all countries
and suggests that, in some instances, it is advances
in medical technology that have aggravated the
problems by merely creating a demand for more of the
same instead of stimulating the search for
alternative strategies:

Increased knowledge has often led to too much specialisation in medicine and to the large uncontrolled proliferation and fragmentation of health services. This, in turn, has led many countries to develop what amounts to disintegrated systems of health care dominated entirely by specialists ... Coverage of peoples' health needs has suffered and resources and manpower have been wasted. Worse the public's expectations have constantly grown, influenced often by considerations far removed from those of good health care ... This has meant that health systems have been too much characterised by a hit and run approach ... There are no clear health policies, no effective structures for health planning and no adequate system for assessing the real value of new development plans or how they are put into effect.

THE THEORETICAL BACKGROUND

Routine data collection is generally associated with the analyses of 'the public health' and with measuring overall improvements in the state of the nation's health. For this purpose, there are two basic requirements, a detailed and accurate description of the population and a measure of health or disease. A census has been carried out in Great Britain every ten years since 1801 except in 1941 when it was suspended during the Second World War. Following an Act of Parliament in 1836, provision was made for the registration of births and deaths and this was made compulsory in 1874. This laid the basis of the present system with mortality data as the principal measure of health or ill health ofa population. The various measures are discussed further in the next chapter. The use of mortality data can be illustrated by the evidence in the Black Report (Department of Health and Social Security, 1980) on social inequalities and health:

1. Children born into unskilled manual workers' families are 4 times more likely to die in the first years of life than those born into professional families.
2. Boys in unskilled workers' families are twice as likely to die between 1 and 14 years of age as boys in professional families (girls are 1½ times as likely to

die).

3. Unskilled male workers are 2½ times as likely to die between the ages of 15 and 14 as professionals.

4. A child born to professional parents is likely to live over 5 years longer than a child born into the family of an unskilled manual labourer.

The limitations of mortality as an indicator of chronic illness have been recognised and although data on morbidity are less comprehensive and more difficult to collect, their importance in planning for health service provision is evident. Again their contribution can be illustrated with reference to social inequalities in health. Based on the General Household Survey (1983) and considering both acute and chronic illness, the higher socio-economic groups report less of both types of illness. In 1981 9 per cent of males and 12 per cent of females in professional families reported restricted activity due to acute illness compared with 12 per cent of males and 17 per cent of females in unskilled manual workers' families. Chronic illness was reported by 10 per cent of professionals (males and females) compared with 19 per cent of males and 31 per cent of females in unskilled manual workers.

In the heyday of public health, national and local reports commented on the state of the public health and this enabled a regular review of the effect of public health measures and indicated priorities for action. In Britain, medical officers of health produced an Annual Report on the health of the town or county although these ceased in the 1970's with the demise of the position of Medical Officer of Health. An annual statement on the National Health which is produced by the Department of Health continues to the present. The growth of nationalised health services, the increased commitment of central funds and academic developments in epidemiology and health care planning led to further refinement of the health care planning process and the systems that were developing.

As Knox (1979) noted, planning for health care cannot be divorced from the wider aspects of planning and most models use a cybernetic planning cycle.

The focal point of planning is the act of choosing between alternative means towards desired ends. In individuals this is seen simply as rational behaviour. Social planning, by analogy, may be seen as rational behaviour among groups and communities. It is the process through which collective goals are pursued and appropriate methods agreed. Health planning, and within it, health care planning, are subsets of this process.

Inherent in this system is a definition of the problem, an assessment or measurement of its extent, severity, course and impact on the community and, a commitment to evaluation which may be limited to the achievement of criteria representing established norms or guidelines. Although the concept of health indicators had existed for many years (Stouman and Falk, 1936) the 1970's saw a rapid development and by 1981 in a publication based on a number of European Workshops, held between 1979 and 1981, Culyer (1981) was able to produce:

... a source book that will not only introduce those who are unfamiliar with it to the field, but indicate the directions taken, problems tackled, and solutions to practical problems, offered, by current research in health indicators. The comprehensive bibliography and detailed country-by-country data sources will be useful to those concerned with research in health indicators whether as 'customers' or as 'suppliers' of research.

This comprehensive volume included economic measures, but these will not be examined further here. Health indicators can be grouped into three main categories:

1. Indicators of health status of individuals in a community. These include mortality, morbidity, disability, absence from work or perceived health. Virtually all of these health status indicators measure departures from health.
2. Indicators of the work, scope and efficiency of health care services. This includes the bulk of the routine hospital and community statistics, treated episodes of illness, number of clinics, staff contacts and procedures carried out. Measures of the availability, acc-essibility and acceptabiliy of health

services can also be included.

3. Indicators of the social or environmental status of the community which relate to health. These may be regarded as a measure or indicator of the risk to the individual in a community such as environmental pollution, overcrowding in houses, passive smoking or a measure of social class or unemployment.

It should be noted that (1) and (3) may reflect the need of a community or may be used to measure the impact of health care. Similarly, (2) may be used to indicate perceived needs of a community - their presentation to health care forming a consultation rate - or it may indicate the number and availability of doctors in a particular clinic.

Paradoxically, some of the very changes which encouraged theoretical developments hindered the establishment of effective health information systems for planning, evaluation and the determination of priorities. The establishment of the practice of community medicine was in essence founded on the approach of its basic disciplines of epidemiology, planning, management, social sciences and statistics, and aimed to provide a health service research and intelligence function. However, in most health authorities in Britain, this failed to take place. Lack of recruitment, small under-resourced departments, a separation between the academic and service components and a resistance by the health service meant that little was achieved. Instead of combining the best of the former practices of public health, medical administration and social medicine it tended in many instances to get submerged by trivia and instead of being an active and progressive influence became largely reactive. Although community medicine may have failed to live up to the initial expectations, the theory and application of planning for health care has now become more established within the National Health Service at national, regional and district levels and this will be discussed briefly with special emphasis on the district level. The wider international perspective will be considered towards the end of the chapter.

PLANNING AND INFORMATION IN A HEALTH SERVICE

One of the main encouragements to a critical examination of the current information system is a change in philosophy within the system. Since the 1960's a number of changes have been proposed which have made it apparent that there is insufficient information available to assess the effectiveness of existing health care; whether or not it was meeting need and which alternative forms of provision were or should be more effective and efficient.

Traditionally, much information from health services has been associated with process, that is, the work carried out, perhaps because it is the simplest to collect and justifies staff by indicating their work load. Typically, reports will contain tables showing the number of school medicals carried out, the number of patients attending a clinic or the number of elderly visited at home by a health visitor. Such accounting gives no indication of the outcome of such procedures, any resulting improvement in health or the quality of the care achieved. Records of immunisations performed are perhaps one of the few examples where process can be assumed to have a reasonable relationship to an outcome - that is, an immune state. There is in general, however, little indication of the population at risk, the varying need of those attending or the outcome of many traditional health care practices.

In Britain during the 1960's and 1970's, a number of reports, surveys and government documents encouraged a change in emphasis from hospital to community care (Department of Health and Social Security, 1976; Department of Health and Social Security, 1977). More recently the DHSS document Health Care and its Costs (1983) identified new policies of community care which had been designed to accelerate the transfer of patients and resources from hospital to the community. While most people (professionals and public) would sympathise with the trend to provide good community care rather than the traditional form of care in large institutions, it is necessary to examine the quality of care that is achieved particularly in relation to costs.

In the 1980's, there has been a renewed emphasis in the National Health Service on management responsibility, clinical budgeting and control of costs within the service resulting in the abolition of area health authorities in 1982

Planning for Health and Resource Allocation

(Department of Health and Social Security, 1979) and
a further reorganisation in 1984 following the
Griffiths Report (1983). Prior to this it had been
recognised that allocation of resources within the
health service had not occurred in the most rational
fashion: it could perhaps best be described as
giving resources to maintain services that already
existed. In 1975, the Secretary of State for Social
Services appointed the Resource Allocation Working
Party (RAWP) with the aim of establishing a system
for distributing resources which would be
'responsive objectively, equitably and efficiently
to relative need'. The only easily available
measure of need was mortality and this was adopted
by the Working Party as the weighting system for
financial allocations. Mortality rates were then
related to such factors as population, patient flows
and different types of service provision such as
out-patients, in-patients, community services etc
(Department of Health and Social Security, 1976).
    Initially, this attempt to relate resources to
need was welcomed, particularly by those regional
health authorities who were considered to have under
provision and hence anticipated some funds becoming
available for new developments. Anxiety was
expressed by those authorities who were deemed to
have over provision and whose resources were to be
cut progressively. This was true especially of
inner London and doubts were voiced about the best
methods of allocating resources within regions to
take account of differing need. It was suggested
that in areas of social deprivation, standardised
mortality ratios did not reflect the burden of
chronic illness or the impact of such illness on
health services. Although some regions with health
districts in inner London have developed a further
weighting system which takes account of social
deprivation, others have not. This additional
weighting system is crude and is based on three
factors.

1. The percentage of New Commonwealth
   immigrants.
2. The percentage of households lacking the
   use of a basic amenity.
3. The percentage of pensioners living
   alone.

With special reference to London (Greater London
Council, 1985) it was noted that the resulting
system did not deal with:

1. The redistribution from high technology care to services for chronic illness.
2. The inequalities in health between social classes.

Just at the time that pressure from professionals, health authorities and planners was mounting for a review of the RAWP system to take account by some means of social deprivation and chronic illness, the recommendations of the Korner Committee (1982) and the detailed reports on different parts of the service which followed, proposed a complete overhaul of the national provision of health information.

Recognising the key position of District Health Authorities, Korner proposed a system based on a minimum data set. This was considered to be the data without which a health authority and its management team would be handicapped in the discharge of their duty to plan, monitor and account for the services for which they were responsible. It was recognised that such a data set might not be sufficient for all purposes at local level, but when aggregated would provide appropriate information at regional and national levels for managing the health services.

The Korner Committee suggested that data are collected for the following reasons:

1. Planning and monitoring.
2. Evaluation and research.
3. Operational control.
4. Treatment of individual patients.
5. Legal requirements.
6. Accountability.

The committee concentrated on (1), (2) and (4), but the present general concern for information has meant that other bodies, professional groups, researchers and the public have contributed to and widened the debate. Attention has been drawn to the virtual total lack of information on the work of general practitioners and the relationship between the Family Practitioner Committees (which became independent authorities in 1985) and District Health Authorities (Department of Health and Social Security, 1984).

The Korner view is that data on services provided should be matched against a projected and an actual budget as well as against a target population, so that estimates may be made of the cost of the services and the coverage achieved.

Linked to this is the proposal that with community activities there should be a grouping under programmes such as immunisation or health promotion and although it will be possible to determine the differing health professionals contributing, the aim will be rather to assess the activity in relation to client groups, for example, pre-school children or elderly persons, rather than to obtain a picture of the overall work of health visitors.

Information is data meaningful to the recipient. Thus to become information, data normally have to be collected, processed, analysed and presented to satisfy a defined need. Information should have the capacity to make the recipient review his options and where appropriate, change his course of action.

(Converting data into Information - report from the Korner committee).

Both the Korner and Griffiths reports have emphasised the importance of well designed and comprehensive information systems for the planning and evaluation of health services. The existing forms of data collection are inefficient, patchy, incomplete and not well used and this cycle means that neither those who collect the data nor those who would wish to use it feel that the work is worthwhile. Indeed, this very separation into those who collect and those who seek to use data illustrates a fundamental problem. It is generally accepted that unless those who collect data for management of health services can also make use of the information themselves to review and plan their own clinical care, then it is unlikely that these data will be efficiently collected. In addition, health authorities now recognise the importance of turning data into information and the need for its suitable presentation to those involved in health care. As a result, many districts are now employing information officers and developing multi-disciplinary teams with a major contribution coming from epidemiologists, community medicine practitioners, demographers and other social scientists. The Korner and Griffiths reports have called for the development of new measures to examine the efficiency of health care with the emphasis on outcome rather than process measures. However, less attention has been paid to the virtual absence of data on health needs and outcomes, in terms of improved health at the individual level.

The need for action in district health authorities is summed up in the following extract from a health authority document:

> Use of information in this authority has remained, on the whole, confined to annual planning exercises and surveys, when broadly based crude averages are employed and attention is focused on developments and cuts at the margin rather than at the bulk of resources used and services provided. Much of the information collected is never analysed, and little of it is used for day-to-day management. Because of years of under-use, information systems have become less reliable and accurate. Nor can existing data be linked together in a consistent and uniform way so as to establish the vital communication between what the authority is doing for its patients and resources employed to do it. The recent arrival of severe financial constraints, allocations based on population and the demand for managerial accountability has necessitated changes of attitude, techniques and management styles. Information is now recognised as being required at all levels for planning, decision making and action, and data must therefore have qualities of accuracy, timeliness and relevancy.

At local level, information can be divided into three broad categories:

1. <u>Management Information</u>. Currently most of the data collected in the NHS fall into this category. It includes data on manpower, admissions, deaths and discharges, waiting lists, clinic attendances, clinics held and procedures such as immunisation that have been carried out. It is based on the returns of health service employees and is collected to provide information for the authority. Demographic data are also used in management and planning but usually 'comes down' to health authorities although some may be derived from local patient registers.

2. <u>Personal Information</u>. This includes patient records, indices of 'at risk'

groups and care groups kept by health personnel. Some management information is derived from this and indeed, the actual records often contain information which, if recorded in a suitable format, could be used in management and planning to assess need and outcome. Currently review groups are comparing existing data collection with what would be required when the Korner recommendations are implemented and although some new categories of information will be necessary, much will simply need to be collated and recorded more systematically.

3. Qualitative Information. This is often thought of as 'knowledge' and is seldom recorded or available in an organised manner. Patients and professionals have difficulty in finding out what local services exist - both statutory and voluntary - what types of help or advice are offered, how long patients have to wait or what new developments may assist patients with particular needs.

At present most data flows from the bottom of the health service to the top and data are often collected only with the objective of providing information for planning and managing the health service. While this will undoubtedly continue there is the requirement for local information to be locally available and locally exchanged. The Minister of Health has stated that 'District Health Authorities will have to ensure that their plans really do encompass health services as a whole and not just those under their immediate control.'
As a result of these reports, and economic pressures on health care services unprecedented effort is being devoted to a complete review of information within the National Health Service in order to construct a system that should lead to improved care for the patient and provide more effective information for those with responsibility for managing the different levels of the service. In complement to improved systems of electronic monitoring and clinic and ward based computer systems as well as computers in general practice, there is a requirement for major new initiatives in three fields:

1. A unique patient number.

2. New measures of socio-economic or social deprivation.
3. New measures of health status to assess need and outcome.

The aim would be to have a unique number for every patient which would enable all contacts with the health service, general medical practitioner, consultant, community clinic, health service laboratory or radiology department, accident and emergency department, outpatient or inpatient departments to be linked easily. This would require a single system acceptable to the Family Practitioner Services and the District Health Authorities. While a unified system would be essential in defined local areas, to be fully effective, a nationally accepted system would be required to take account of patients attending hospitals or clinics in different districts and of migration within the country. Although there has been interest in unique patient numbers and record linkage for many years, practice has been limited to a few experimental areas. However the possibility of a national system is now under active discussion (Baldwin and Gill, 1982).

A combined approach by Family Practitioner Services and District Health Authorities should be able to produce a master patient index which can then be related to districts, family practitioner services or an individual general practice list (Department of Health and Social Security, 1985). The unique number proposed for this record linkage should be automatically generated from the patient's name, date of birth and sex and thus would not be dependent on any of the diverse existing numbering systems. All health professionals and patients would have to assume a new responsibility for accurate data generation.

The Korner report has recommended the inclusion of 'place of residence' code in all Family Practitioner Service records. If the use of postcode were adopted throughout, then individual data could be aggregated for enumeration districts, wards and districts. Confidentiality would have to be ensured although unless information is exchanged about people receiving care from different sections of service, for example, cervical cytology screening, it is not possible to identify those who are not receiving a service and who may be at greatest risk.

Postcodes are the basis for the ACORN

classification of neighbourhoods which is a
relatively new system of breaking down a district
into small areas of similar social characteristics.
(CACI, undated). Although originally developed for
marketing purposes, it may have a value in studies
of social deprivation and health and may prove to be
a useful indicator of need. With increasing
problems in the use of traditional measures of
social class, due to high unemployment, a more
elderly population and the limitations of using
husbands' social class, a new measure such as ACORN
which can be applied to all may prove to be an
additional tool in planning. A number of studies
(Morgan and Chinn, 1983; Curtis and Woods,
1983) are examining its role, but further work is
required to determine its relationship to existing
indicators of health and the feasibility of its
application to population studies.

Recognising the diversities within an average
health district of 300,000 - 500,000 people the use
of smaller defined areas for certain purposes has
been proposed (King and Court, 1984).

> Care in the community is the message of the
> eighties. But to move in the new direction
> we need fresh attitudes and different
> styles in planning ... and put simply
> locality planning taps knowledge of local
> need through local people - priorities and
> solutions are locally derived.

The authors showed that the use of data from small
locally defined communities led to a redistribution
of facilities and staff and a change of attitude:

> ... for the health authority regards itself as
> bringing a contribution of service to the
> community to be used in conjunction with all
> its other medley of services.

These developments may lead to better ways of
identifying patients, of defining populations and
describing individual or community social
characteristics but it is necessary to examine the
purpose of health care before considering the
measures of health status which may be used to
assess need and outcome.

HEALTH CARE - WHAT ARE THE OBJECTIVES?

Equality is a term often used in discussions on
health care and there is an assumption that equity
is an objective of the National Health Service, but
it is essential to be clear what is supposed to be
equal. Considerable work on this subject has been
carried out by health economists. Le Grand (1982)
proposed five concepts of equality which should be
considered for any public services:

1. Equality of public expenditure - this
   proposes that imbalances between the
   regions, for example in hospital
   specialties, should be rectified.
2. Equality of final income - this proposes
   that public expenditure on any particular
   service should be allocated to favour the
   poor.
3. Equality of use - this proposes that
   amounts of service used should be
   equalised.
4. Equality of cost - this proposes that all
   individuals face the the same private cost
   per unit of service used.
5. Equality of outcome - this proposes that
   everyone should end up with equal status
   of health.

West (1981) considers that equity can be
viewed as having two possible dimensions.

1. Equal treatment of equals - horizontal
   equity. This seeks to provide the same
   amount of health care for individuals who
   are identified in terms of all
   relevant characteristics such as health
   status, age, sex, geographical location
   etc.
2. Unequal treatment of unequals - vertical
   equity. It is necessary to quantify the
   degree of inequality that exists and to
   establish a relationship between the level
   of health status and the level of service
   that should be received. It is not enough
   to say that those with worse health status
   should receive more health care, it is
   necessary to take account of how much
   additional health care those who are worse
   off should receive.

At the thirtieth session of the Regional
Committee of Member States of the World Health
Organisation European Region in 1980, the first
common health policy was approved - the European
Strategy for attaining health for all (World Health
Organisation, 1984).

The first aim is to ensure 'equity in health'
between and within countries, initially by reducing
differences in health levels between countries and
between different population groups within
countries by at least 25 per cent by the year 2000.
This called for a fundamental reorientation of
countries' health developments and outlined four
main areas of concern: lifestyle and health; risk
factors affecting health and the environment;
reorientation of the health care system itself; and
finally, the political, managerial, technological,
manpower, research and other support services
necessary to bring about the desired changes in
these areas. The strategy urged that a much higher
priority be given to health promotion and disease
prevention; that not merely the health services but
all sectors with an impact on health should take
positive steps to monitor and improve it; that much
more emphasis should be placed on the role that
individuals, families and communities can play in
health development; and finally, that primary health
care should be the major approach to bring about
these changes.

This represented a landmark in health
development among the European peoples. Never
before had the countries of the Region agreed to
adopt a single health policy on a common basis for
subsequent developments, both in individual member
states and in the Region as a whole. This was
followed by a commitment to review their health
developments, bringing their health policies and
programming in line with the health for all strategy
and, by systematic monitoring and submission of a
report every second year, ensure that concrete
action was taking place.

To assist in this, 38 Regional targets have
been defined and a set of regional indicators have
been devised. One essential for this is an
efficient information system. WHO notes many of the
proposed indicators are already part of the
information system for most countries and that data
on others are often available from existing
reporting systems or summaries in health and related
sectors. Some indicators call for special data
collection through sample surveys. WHO also

33

indicate that further studies are required to refine the list of indicators, especially those related to disability, health promotion and environmental health.

General practice perhaps best illustrates the possibility of bringing together the individual and collective approach. In 1977 the Leeuwenhorst Working Party (Royal College of General Practitioners, 1977) in considering the special function of the general practitioner extended the concept to 'personal, primary and continuing care to individuals, families and a practice population'. This recognition of responsibility towards individuals and defined populations relates to the concept of anticipatory care (Royal College of General Practitioners, 1981) which brings together prevention and care.

There is a combined approach to caring for the ill patient and simultaneously seeking, through a variety of means, to encourage health in the future. Individual care is combined with the epidemiological approach to communities.

Just as there is a need to measure health status, it is also necessary to recognise that the allocation of resources designed to improve health may not lie solely within the NHS. While a major responsibility of caring for the sick must lie with the health services, many of the factors that influence health are related to the environment, education, poverty or unemployment and much of the allocation of resources that may lead to an improvement of health lie outside the health service.

Most of the discussion in this chapter has related to routine data but it is important to realise that routine data may require to be enriched for special purposes or supplemented by specially collected data from surveys or detailed analyses of data collected for other purposes such as clinical care. Cartwright (1983) has provided a thorough review of health surveys which illustrates the importance of the partnership of research workers with those in health authorities who are involved in the preparation of routine data sets.

Thus decisions need to be made - what can be measured?; what kind of health measures for what kind of purpose?; what needs to be routinely available and what collected specially?; what kind of system can provide better information for individual health care and for planning and managing health services?

REFERENCES

Baldwin, J.A. and Gill, L.E. (1982) 'The District Number: A Comparative Test of some Record Matching Methods', Comm Med, 4, 265-275

CACI, ACORN, A Classification of Residential Neighbourhoods, developed by CACI, London (no date)

Cartwright, A. (1983) Health Surveys in Practice and Potential, King's Fund, London

Culyer, A.J. (1981) Health and Health Indicators. Proceedings of a European Workshop, Report to the British Social Science Research Council and the European Science Foundation, University of York

Curtis, S. and Woods, K. (1983) The Local Morbidity Survey as a Health Planning Instrument, paper presented at the King's Fund Centre, Need for Health Services in London

Department of Health and Social Security (1976) Priorities for Health and Social Services in England, HMSO, London

Department of Health and Social Security (1977) The Way Forward, HMSO, London

Department of Health and Social Security (1976) Sharing Resources for Health in England, Report of the Resource Allocation Working Party, HMSO, London

Department of Health and Social Security (1979) Patients First, Consultation Paper on the Structure and Management of the National Health Service in England and Wales, HMSO, London

Department of Health and Social Security (1980) Inequalities in Health: A Report of a Research Working Group, HMSO, London

Department of Health and Social Security (1983) Health Care and its Costs, HMSO, London

Department of Health and Social Security (1984) Report of the Joint Working Group on Collaboration between Family Practitioner Committees and District Health Authorities, Chairman Mrs P. Petrine, HMSO, London

Department of Health and Social Security (1985) Results of a Study into the Data required to support the Exchange of Information between Family Practitioner Services and Hospital and Community Health Services, Report by Arthur Anderson and Co, HMSO, London

Greater London Council (1984) A Critical Guide to Health Services Resource Allocation in London, GLC, London

Griffiths, E.R. (1983) Report of the NHS Management Enquiry, HMSO, London

King, D. and Court, M. (1984) 'A Sense of Scale', Hlth Soc Serv J, June 21, 734

Knox, E.G. (1979) Epidemiology in Health Care Planning, Oxford University Press, Oxford

Leeuwenhorst Working Party (1977) J Roy Coll Gen Pract, 27, 117

Le Grand, J. (1982) The Strategy of Equality, Allen and Unwin, London

Morgan, M. and Chinn, S. (1983) 'ACORN Group, Social Class and Child Health', J of Epidem Comm Hlth, 37, 196-203

Office of Population Censuses and Surveys (1983) General Household Survey 1981, HMSO, London

O'Neill P. (1983) Health Crisis 2000, published for WHO, Heinemann Medical Books Ltd, pp. 5-6, London

Royal College of General Practitioners, (1981) Health and Prevention in Primary Care, (Report from General Practice No. 18), RCGP, London

Steering Group on Health Services Information (1982) First Report to the Secretary of State, (Chairman Mrs E. Korner), HMSO, London

Stouman, K. and Falk, I.S. (1936) 'Health Indices: A Study of Objective Indices of Health in Relation to Environment and Sanitation', Bulletin of Health of the League of Nations, 8, 63-69

West, P.A. (1981) 'Theoretical and Practical Equity in the National Health Service in England', Soc Sci Med, 15c, 117-122

White, K.L. (1974) 'Contemporary Epidemiology', Int J Epidem, 3, 295-303

World Health Organisation (1984) Regional Targets in Support of the Regional Strategy for Health for All, EUR/RC34/7 Rev 1 6388D/6389D, Regional Office for Europe, WHO, Copenhagen

World Health Organisation (1984) Proposed Plan of Action for the Implementation of the Regional Strategy for Attaining Health for All by the Year 2000, EUR/RC34/14 6765L, Regional Office for Europe, WHO, Copenhagen

World Health Organisation (1984) List of Proposed Indicators for Monitoring Progress towards Health for All in the European Region, EUR/RC34/13 4762D/2650D, Regional Office for Europe, WHO, Copenhagen

Chapter 3.

MEASURING HEALTH STATUS

Clearly, attempts to measure health status must be founded in some concept of what constitutes health, or those conditions, signs and experiences which might indicate ill-health. Thus health measurement is inevitably tied to two interlinked issues: how 'health' is defined and the purpose for which the measurement is required. As we have seen there are three concepts which dominate this field: health, disease and illness. Each of these can be said to incorporate biological, psychological and social factors, but each implies a different emphasis. The most intractable of these concepts from a measurement point of view is 'health', since although there is at least some agreement on 'not-health', there is virtually none on 'health' or the even vaguer notion of well-being. From a medical point of view, the increasing sophistication of technology facilitates diagnosis in microsystems of the human body, pinpointing small deviations from 'normal' functioning which would, hitherto, have been undetectable by the most talented clinician or by the patient. In fact, few people would be declared totally healthy from a biological perspective. Thus the presence of health relates to social, psychological, physical and functional capacities in a manner relative to time, place and contemporary technology.

Disease is much easier to classify, although it should be noted that some 50 per cent of patients present themselves for consultation with clusters of symptoms which cannot be found in the International Classification of Diseases. Nevertheless, there is considerable consensus on what constitutes disease, although some maladies, as we shall note in chapter 8, are culture specific. Disease and disability imply the presence of signs and symptoms susceptible to classification by the prevailing system; measurement, therefore, tends to be based upon the incidence and prevalence of morbidity, symptoms and, of course, mortality.

Illness has a very definite subjective component. One may be 'diseased' and not ill, ill but not 'diseased', since illness involves changes in the individual's experience of his or her mental, physical and/or social being. The perception of such changes will depend upon many factors which are not constant over time, for example, current activities and the degree to which the individual is absorbed in them; background 'noise', that is, the extent of pre-existing discomfort to which a person has become accustomed; the expectations and demands related to social and occupational roles; the costs and benefits of a declaration and/or diagnosis of illness. Indeed, it could be argued that one of the functions of a general practitioner is to help people 'decide', in some sense, whether or not to become ill. Therefore the assessment of illness would certainly involve some subjective component relating to comparative perception. Where health status is to be defined by degree of disability or functional capacity the implications will differ in relation to the physical and social requirements of the individual's daily activities. For example, in some subsistence societies people manage to function quite well in spite of suffering from endemic conditions such as schistosomiasis, which might severely disrupt the activities of a worker in an industrialised society. Similarly, within cultures, different groups, the young and old, the single and married, female and male will suffer somewhat different consequences from an impairment in their usual functioning. On the whole, it can be said that the more varied the circumstances and the populations in which a health indicator will be used, the more general it should be. Thus measures range from the highly specific, for example, assessment of the degree of breathlessness in heart disease, to the very general, for example, psychological well-being.

The purpose for which health assessment is undertaken will influence the form of the resulting instrument. Economists are eager to have a single global index which can be computed from valuations of states of health and which can be incorporated into analyses of costs versus outcome. This index could then be used for the determination of priorities for the allocation of scarce resources.

Clinicians, conversely, are more interested in health profiles which give a more comprehensive picture of individual patterns and changes in health status.

Currently, many different types of health measurements and indicators are in use and it would be impossible to review them all. The rest of this chapter will describe some examples from the range available.

MORTALITY RATES

Mortality rates have the advantage of being routinely collected and easily available in many countries and are now, in Great Britain, used as a basis for resource allocation in the health service (Department of Health and Social Security, 1976).

In poorer countries where deaths from infections and parasitic diseases are still common and where infant and maternal mortality rates are high, information on cause and number of deaths is very useful both as a measure of the overall health status of the country and as a basis for planning and priority setting. However, in more affluent societies, mortality rates are gradually losing favour. As longevity increases it becomes more difficult to diagnose cause of death unequivocally because of the rise in chronic multicausal disease and disability. This means that both general and disease specific rates become less useful. Moreover, the death rate for some conditions, for example, maternal mortality, is now so low that annual rates are subject to large and artificial fluctuations rendering them useless for practical purposes. In addition, thresholds of acceptability tend to change as expectations rise. Thus, the seriousness with which a particular mortality statistic is regarded could increase at the same time as the rate is decreasing. A low perinatal mortality rate may mean more survivors at risk. Objections have also been expressed to the implicit assumption made by the users of mortality rates that all deaths are basically of equal importance. The distinction has been made between avoidable and unavoidable deaths (Rutstein, Berenberg, Chalmers, Fishman, Perrin and Zuidema, 1980) and focus placed on 'unnecessary untimely mortality' which might be avoided by adequate primary prevention. A further limitation of mortality rates as a basis for planning health services in industrialised countries is that they emphasise quantity rather than quality of life. Chronic illness and disability impose much more of a drain on resources than outright death. Improved mortality rates do not necessarily imply a generally improved health status (at least within countries) since the reality may be that fewer people are dying, but survivors are experiencing increased morbidity. An analysis of routine statistics for Great Britain on deaths under the age of one year, showed that socio-demographic factors explained four times as much of the variance between cases as did medical care (Martini, Allan, Davison and Backett, 1979). This highlights the fact that traditional measures such as mortality are now insufficiently sensitive to be useful in the evaluation of health and medical services. However, mortality rates continue to be appropriate in providing information on the natural history and treatment of disease and in facilitating comparative analysis of group and geographic differences, such as, death by occupational group and the well-known gradient of mortality from the south to the north of Great Britain.

MORBIDITY MEASURES

Morbidity rates, although they reflect the wider effects of disease, have the disadvantage of being less readily available and subject to considerable variation in quality. Attempts to improve the quality and accuracy of morbidity statistics have developed in a number of ways:

1. Refined indices, such as incidence and prevalence rates for specific conditions, absence from work, episodes of illness and type and duration of disability.

2. Disability indices, which assess the degree to which people are able to perform the essential tasks of daily life.

3. Symptom or function indices, which focus on clinical symptoms, on the ability to function in social and occupational roles and on the capacity to carry out selected behaviours. They may also assess the effect of illness or disability on a variety of social, domestic and personal activities. Reports may be made by observers or by the persons themselves. Such indices include subjective measures

which attempt to tap the daily experience of distress as perceived by the individuals concerned.

Most of these indicators note departures from 'normal' functioning, or the presence of symptoms and signs of disease or malaise, since it has proved much easier to express, record and quantify departures from health rather than to find indices of health itself (however defined). Such measures may be kept routinely - as in hospital activities analysis, or be incorporated into special surveys and studies.

REFINED INDICES

Measuring the prevalence and incidence of disease has the advantage of breaking general morbidity into more manageable chunks to which specific policies and treatments can be directed and evaluated. However, it necessitates the drawing together of data from different sources; hospital records, registers, case reports and surveillance systems. This collation requires considerable epidemiological skill in the extrapolation of data, allowing for incomplete figures and adjusting for differences in the diagnosis of related diseases. Routinely kept statistics may be supplemented by periodic surveys of randomly selected members of the population.

Incidence and prevalence figures are, perforce, biased and incomplete and require that individuals come to the notice of the health system in some way. A great deal of minor illness is undoubtedly missed for this reason, although the common cold, for example, is a major cause of absence from work and consequent loss of productivity. Other indices in this category include hospital bed days, sickness absence from work and number of prescriptions issued. Such measures do give a rough guide to the health status of a population or community but are inflated by utilisation for non-medical reasons, or give underestimates because of the failure of affected persons to come to the notice of the recording system.

DISABILITY INDICES

A distinction has been made between impairment, disability and handicap (Harris, 1971) where impairment refers to some physiological condition such as a crippled limb, partial hearing or blindness; disability is the degree to which this affects the functioning of the individual - some impairments may be minimal in their impact because of 41 technical aids; handicap represents the extent to which the impairment interferes with occupational and social activities. Although they are referred to as disability measures, most instruments incorporate all three of these distinctions, without necessarily making them explicit. Typically they include the notions of physical and social incapacity in relation to a variety of activities. Levels of disability can be used as indicators of the severity of particular diseases and the outcome of treatment, as well as giving a guide to the potential demand for services. Where the main health problems of a country are chronic diseases, disability indices are more helpful tools for evaluation than are cure rates or mortality figures.

The incorporation of disability measures into special surveys commonly focuses upon the respondent's experience of limitations to 'usual activities' in recent weeks, confinement to bed or days lost from work or school. Strictly speaking these are assessments of handicap, rather than disability per se and may not be useful as descriptors of long-term illness or impairment.

One of the best known and oldest of the disability scales is the Activities of Daily Living (ADL) index developed by Katz, Ford, Moskowitz, Jacobson and Jaffee (1963). This index was constructed for evaluating treatment in relation to specific groups and thus focuses upon disabilities relevant to those groups. Independence and adequacy in bathing, toileting, dressing, feeding, etc. of patients are rated on ordinal scales by observers. Scores are summed to give a single total. ADL scores have been shown to be predictive of outcome in stroke and hip fracture (Katz, Ford, Heiple and Newill, 1964; Katz, Ford, Chinn and Newill, 1966). This index appears to be very useful with a restricted range of patients. However, the range of handicaps and their sequelae tapped by the instrument is by no means comprehensive and the populations with which it might be used are necessarily restricted. The use of a single index inevitably means a loss of information about variability, because different patterns of restriction, with somewhat different implications, can be reduced to the same score.

A more recent instrument developed in Great Britain uses Guttman scaling, a technique which assumes that disabilities can be ordered. For example, 7 disabilities always score worse than 6 and a score of 7 would assume that items 1-6 had also been affirmed. It is claimed that the scale can be 42 used to predict the next stage in the progression of a disease. Items include questions on housework, dressing, hygiene and physical mobility (Williams, Johnston, Willis and Bennett, 1976). The activities making up the scale do not form a complete description of the activities of daily living, but the instrument has the advantage of having two scales, one for men and one for women and work is still proceeding to develop and refine the scale further.

Two scales designed specifically for arthritis sufferers are the Health Assessment Questionnaire (HAQ) and the Arthritis Impact Measurement Scales (AIMS). The HAQ has 21 questions with 9 components and each question can be scored on a scale of 1 to 3. Items include dressing and grooming, getting up, eating, walking, reach, personal hygiene, gripping and grasp. These items are self-administered and correlate with observed patient performance in the range 0.47 to 0.88 which is not particularly high (Fries, Spitz and Young, 1982). The AIMS has 49 items which are summed into 9 scales, indexed 0-10 from minimum to maximum disability. The scales include questions on dexterity, household activities, pain, social activities, depression and anxiety as well as activities of daily living. Scores are said to correlate highly with physician judgements and standard measures of physical function (Meenan, Gertman and Mason, 1980). The specificity of these two instruments makes them unsuitable for use with groups other than the chronically ill and their validity and reliability are not yet well established.

A scale based on a more general definition of disability at low levels is a 30 item scale developed by McDowell and Roberts (1983). The items reflect physical, mental and social well-being and positive concepts of health. However, the items have been selected from a variety of other questionnaires and item analysis for the choice of the final content was on the basis of 'expert review'. Consequently, it may be more reflective of professional opinions about low-level disability than those of lay people and its use should be restricted to situations where this is appropriate.

A group in London has produced a single measure of health status based upon 29 combinations of disability and distress, using descriptions obtained from doctors and nurses. Evaluations of eight states of disability and four of severity (including death) have been obtained from health professionals and patients by the use of lengthy interviews. The authors claim the scale obtained is a ratio scale and that it yields a single score which can be used as an indicator of hospital performance, where changes in health status can be linked to costs of care and treatment (Rosser and Kind, 1978). This scale certainly has potential as a measure of the outcome of hospitalisation. Unfortunately the small number of subjects involved in valuation casts doubt upon the validity of the scale, particularly (as the authors admit) since there were wide individual differences. Another problem is that the scale assumes health states to be either permanent or of indefinite duration. This scale would appear to need a great deal more groundwork on its validity and reliability before it can be regarded as a credible tool.

An advantage of disability measurements is that people can be graded by degree of limitation rather than simply having or not having some problem, but it should be borne in mind that measures of disability always relate to some culturally-specific assumptions about what constitutes a 'normal' range of abilities and activities. Not only culture, but age, sex, social roles and expectations will have a bearing on the kind and level of activities deemed reasonable by both lay-people and professionals, and, therefore, the extent to which handicap can be supposed to exist.

SYMPTOM AND FUNCTION INDICES

To some extent indicators based upon symptoms and functions cannot be separated from disability indices. There is considerable overlap, with the main distinction being that the latter are somewhat more specialised and narrow in range, whilst the former give a broader picture which may include perceived and experiential elements in psychological and social domains as well as the purely physical and behavioural.

A good example is the Cornell Medical Index (CMI) which is based upon self-report and contains 95 yes-no questions divided into 18 sections referring to physiological disturbance, personal habits, frequency of illness, moods and feelings. Affirmative responses are assumed to indicate some deviation from normal functioning and the total number of 'yes' answers indicates the degree of 'deviancy'. Thus a medically significant emotional disturbance is considered present if the total score is 30 or more, if there are three or more affirmative responses on the psychological section or where four or more questions are not answered or changed. (Brodman, Erdman and Wolff, 1960). The populations upon whom the CMI was standardised are restricted in range and the assumptions about what constitutes normal functioning are based upon a purely medical model.

An assessment instrument for use primarily with the elderly is the Older American's Resources and Services Inventory (OARS) and its shorter version, the Functional Assessment Inventory (Cairl, Pfeiffer, Keller, Burke and Samis, 1983; Fillenbaum and Smyer, 1981). Both instruments have questions relating to mental status, socio-demographic information, mental health, physical health, activities of daily living and the use of social and medical services. Information is obtained by interview. There is also a section to be answered by an informant if the subject is judged to be cognitively incapacitated and scales on which the interviewer rates the patient's impairment in terms of social and financial resources, mental and physical health and daily activities. In addition, the interviewer completes a section concerning his or her judgement of the reliability of the patient's answers. The FAI has 90 less items than the OARS, fewer response categories, a modified coding system and two scales measuring life satisfaction and self-esteem. Although both instruments appear to have face and content validity, discriminant and predictive validity have not been adequately tested. The complexity of the inventory makes it time-consuming to complete and the potential for contradictory information coming from respondent and interviewer is quite large.

Another set of scales developed for clinical assessment, referrals and the epidemiology of geriatric problems represent an Anglo-American enterprise, being based upon information from 445 elderly persons in New York and 396 in London. (Gurland, Kuriansky, Sharpe, Simon, Stiller and Birkett, 1977; Teresi, Golden and Gurland, 1984). The Comprehensive Assessment and Referral Evaluation Scales (CARE) are completed by an informant about the elderly person and tap medical symptoms, such as high blood pressure, shortness of breath, swollen ankles, etc; psychiatric problems, such as trouble in sleeping, loneliness, anxiety, forgetfulness and social problems such as isolation, neighbourhood issues and financial considerations. Construct validation has been established by inter-informant agreement, but grave doubts must be expressed about the appropriateness of some items as indicative of 'problems' and the whole scale is highly dependent upon the judgement of the informant.

An instrument designed to measure general health functioning is the McMaster Health Index Questionnaire (MHIQ) developed in Canada (Chambers, 1982; Chambers, MacDonald, Tugwell, Buchanan and Kraag, 1982). This contains 59 items covering physical mobility, self-care, sight and hearing, general well-being, social and occupational role performance, family support, self-esteem, critical life events, personal relationships and emotional functioning. The questionnaire can be self-completed or administered by an interviewer and all items are phrased in terms of performance on the day of administration of the MHIQ. Content, criterion and construct validity have been assessed in a wide range of patient groups including psychiatric patients, acute care elderly and the chronically ill. The validity of the physical function items is robust but the social and emotional items are considerably weaker. The MHIQ is useful as an adjunct to clinical indicators when used as an assessment of function, and it is simple, acceptable, cheap and reasonably reliable. Its limitations relate mainly to the doubtful validity of many items, although work is proceeding to correct this.

Another instrument which has the advantage of having been designed for both self-administration and interview is the Duke-UNC Health Profile (DUHP), which focuses upon health status in terms of its import to primary care facilities. There are 63 items, 28 of which refer to presence of symptoms and 15 to physical function such as disability days, ambulation and use of upper limbs. There are items on emotional aspects, especially self-esteem and on social function, for example, role performance. This instrument has been validated by comparison tests with other questionnaires and its high reported validity is not surprising in view of the similarity of its items to those in the other instruments used. A test against 'real life' criteria remains to be made and there appears to be uncertainty about temporal consistency (Parkerson, Gehlback, Wagner, James, Clapp and Mulbaier, 1981).

A scale on which a great deal of work has been done in the USA is the Quality of Well-Being Scale (formerly the Index of Well-Being) developed as an instrument for general health policy (Bush, 1984; Kaplan, Bush and Berry, 1976). The Quality of Well-Being (QWB) score combines assessments of quality of life with mortality risk and includes symptom combinations such as pain and shortness of breath with measures of functional ability, social activities, self-care and activities of daily living. A feature of this scale is that functional states are classified according to what a person actually does as opposed to a judgement about capacity. Scores can be expressed as daily profiles on all dimensions as well as by a single comprehensive score. The QWB must be administered by trained interviewers and is very complex, which severely limits its application. Nevertheless, validity and reliability have been extensively tested and appear satisfactory and it is useful as a measure of efficacy and efficiency in health care, allowing output to be related to cost. Therefore, it is most appropriate for clinical trials and the evaluation of medical practices.

A much shorter, simpler index of general health is computed from the Health Perceptions Questionnaire (HPQ) developed by Ware (1976), for the National Centre for Health Services Research in the USA. Here the items consist of statements about personal health to which the person responds in one of five standardised categories on a true-false continuum. These items are then converted into six subscale scores which assess past health, present and future health, health-related worries and concerns, resistance to illness and the tendency to view illness as a part of life. HPQ items are used to compute a General Health Rating Index. The HPQ is self-administered and can also be used in telephone or face-to-face interviews. There is also a version for children. Reliability of the scores is rather low using test-re-test techniques, although internal consistency is high. Validity testing has been based largely on factor analysis and correlations between HPQ scores and other health variables. Some of these correlations proved to be very weak, but further studies are in progress. The Index of General Health has been used to predict utilisation of mental health and medical services and is sensitive to changes in perceived health status. However, it lacks a firm conceptual base and the actual meaning of the scores is quite unclear.

Undoubtedly one of the best products of the health measurement field in the USA has been the Sickness Impact Profile (SIP) developed by a research team in Washington (Bergner, Bobbitt, Pollard, Martin and Gilson, 1976; Bergner, Bobbitt, Carter and Gilson, 1981). The SIP is a questionnaire containing 136 items referring to illness-related dysfunction in 12 domains: work, recreation, emotion, affect, home life, sleep, rest, eating, ambulation, mobility, communication and social interaction. Scores can be in the form of an overall total, or separate for physical and psycho-social areas. The questionnaire may be self-administered or given by a trained interviewer. Several studies have established good convergent and discriminant validity and test-re-test reliability is high. This instrument is suitable for a wide range of patients with acute or chronic conditions and has been used successfully in clinical trials and in surveys of special groups. The SIP is particularly valuable for assessing the impact of illness on the chronically ill and for measuring the effect of non-curative interventions. Its two major limitations are its length and the fact that it can be used only with people who are regarded, or who regard themselves, as ill. A modified version of the SIP called the Functional Limitation Profile was developed at St Thomas', London and adapted for use in Britain where it was used in a study of disabled people in Lambeth (Patrick, Darby, Green, Horton, Locker and Wiggins, 1981). The modification of the items consisted of analysing them for conformity to British usage and rewording them, where necessary, to make them more meaningful to the British population concerned (Patrick, 1981). As will be seen in chapter 8, these rather cursory changes scarcely satisfy the requirements for cross-cultural adaptations and the appropriateness of the Functional Limitation Profile for British samples remains to be established.

Mention should also be made of Langer's Mental Health Scale which was an attempt to produce a short, but reliable means of assessing impairment due to the commoner psychiatric symptoms. The scale items are based on a selection of symptoms taken from the Minnesota Multiphasic Personality Inventory and a neuropsychiatric screening instrument. The 22 items assume unidimensionality and include loss of memory, nervousness, worrying, sleep problems, poor appetite, restlessness, shortness of breath, heart flutters and acid stomach (Langner, 1962). The indiscriminate combining of physical and mental events which are aggregated together in the score and variations by age, sex and socio-economic status which raise issues of the interpretation of group differences pose problems for the validity of this scale.

Few workers in the health indicators field have attempted to construct standardised measures of positive health, presumably for one of two reasons. The first reason is the lack of agreement on the parameters of health as opposed to disease, and the second is the paucity of the English language when it comes to detailing aspects of feeling well as opposed to feeling ill. Two of the better documented attempts both concentrate on mental health, perhaps because psychiatrists and psychologists have been more assured about the features of positive mental health.

An Index of Psychological Well-Being is described by Bradburn (1969). This consists of two scales, one of positive and one of negative affect based upon asking respondents whether, in the past few weeks, they had ever felt bored, restless, excited or interested in something, 'on top of the world', pleased about some accomplishment, depressed, proud at having been complimented and so on.

A similar instrument - the Psychological General Well-Being Index was developed by Dupuy (1974). This index consists of 22 items thought to be representative of six psychological states; anxiety, depression, positive well-being, self-control, general health and vitality. Each item has six response categories according to the intensity or frequency of the experience. Scores can be expressed as totals for each of the subscales or as an overall score. Validity has been tested by correlations with medical history, utilisation of mental health services, psychosomatic complaints and other mental health scales with fairly satisfactory results. However, much of the correlation is explained by the association of negative rather than positive factors. Reliability varies with samples used and has ranged from 0.50 to 0.86 on test-re-test correlation coefficients.

A major drawback of these two instruments is the cultural bias endemic in the assumptions about well-being. American notions of 'feeling good' may well differ considerably from those of a Scotsman or a German. As demonstrated in chapter 8, the use of instruments developed in one society with samples from another culture is usually misleading and always misguided unless further tests of validity and reliability have been carried out in the new context. This is a general problem with all the symptom and functional indicators described. With few exceptions the bulk of work on socio-medical indicators has been carried out in the United States and only the Sickness Impact Profile has been adapted for British use with, as yet, unknown efficacy.

There have been attempts in Britain to develop indicators of disability, functional limitation and general health status. The work of Williams and that of Rosser and Kind has already been described. In addition should be mentioned the work of Hannay and that of Grogono and Woodgate. Hannay, (1978) developed a questionnaire which asks about 44 symptom groups, which refer to feelings rather than disabilities. Administration is by interview and allows subjective responses to items on fatigue, fever, skin trouble, appetite, stomach problems, respiratory problems, general malaise, genito-urinary problems, joint pain, physical mobility and cardiovascular symptoms among others. Items are expressed in non-medical terms and the instrument is probably most useful for assessing patterns of utilisation in general practice and the prevalence of distress in the community. Grogono and Woodgate, (1971) developed an assessment scale for patients where items on work, recreation, physical and mental suffering, communication, sleep, dependency, feeding, excretion and sexual activity are asked by interview and supplemented by observer assessment. Where observations are made by medical staff and students, inter-observer reliability is high (0.88), but test-re-test reliability has not been assessed and the validity is questionable. In addition, the choice of items lacks a rationale. The scale is intended to measure benefit from medical treatment and score can be expressed as health years, or parts thereof, gained as a result of medical intervention, or lost as a result of disease.

A rather more comprehensive instrument is the General Household Survey (GHS) part of which is used routinely to monitor illness episodes, utilisation of health and social services, disability, the effect of illness on people's daily lives and how they cope. The GHS places some emphasis on how people perceive their state of health as well as collecting information on symptoms. Portions of the GHS have been extracted and used as survey instruments, see, for example, Curtis, (1983) and Leavey, (1982). Since its first use by the Office of Population Censuses and Surveys in 1973 several changes have been made to the GHS making assessment of its valdity and reliability difficult (OPCS, 1975-1982). Such analyses as have been done on validity are quite inadequate to give confidence in the meaning and reliability of the data. Respondents are asked a great many questions, some of which are complex, and there is contamination from some questions to others. Therefore, much patience and forebearance is needed by respondents and the instrument is particularly taxing for the old and the ill.

An instrument for the detection of purely psychological problems is the General Health Questionnaire (GHQ) which was developed for community screening by Goldberg (1971). The GHQ (which is misleadingly named) is available in different versions, from 140 items to 12 items and has been found to be effective in detecting the existence of mental problems, although not their severity. Further comments on this questionnaire are made in chapter 5.

The construction of the Nottingham Health Profile, the development of which is fully described in chapter 5, was planned to overcome some of the problems which are evident in most of the instruments described above. It is based upon lay perceptions of health status, thus obviating the need for 'expert' definitions of what exactly it is that constitutes health; it is short and simple; based upon British samples; suitable for clinical or survey work and forms a well validated and reliable measure of 'subjective health' which can be used with a general population as well as with groups of patients. It is appropriate for people who have not been labelled unhealthy and who do not consider themselves to be ill. However, ultimately the NHP, like so many other measures of 'health' came to focus upon negative rather than positive experiences.

THE SEARCH FOR A GLOBAL INDEX

Measures of health status based upon scales and profiles are usually found satisfactory by clinicians, epidemiologists, health researchers and other health professionals. However, economists and those people concerned with health policy and planning have urged the development of single, global indices which would summarise in a single statistic the health status of populations. Such models, typically, assign values to, for example, days of 'health', number of illnesses per annum per person, presumed effects of death, hospital in-patient days and generally involve weightings of the severity of ill health, resulting in a comprehensive index in the form of an annual statistic. An early attempt at this was made by Miller, (1970) with the Q index which was designed for the Indian Health Service in North America to aid policy planning. It is based upon certain assumed values and costs relating to loss of productivity through illness or death, for example, that one hospital in-patient day is equal to a day of premature death; that children of 15 years and under will have 50 years of productive life and that people over the age of 65 years will have six months of productivity ahead of them. Associated numerical values are built into an equation which incorporates crude mortality rate, years of life lost due to premature death, out-patient and in-patient days and days of restricted activities. The resulting statistic is said to indicate population health status and has been used for priority setting in the IHS. However, the somewhat arbitrary assumptions and the bias in valuation of working life makes it only of questionable value in a complex and heterogenous society.

Sullivan (1966; 1971) combined mortality and morbidity in a single score to give a 'life free of disability' index, an extrapolation of life expectancy from which average disability in a lifetime is extracted. The Index assumes all disabilities are equal regardless of their aetiology, type, duration, or effect. Chiang (1965) produced an Index of Health which uses the weighted average mean duration of 'health' of a population per annum, the mean duration of health by age groups and includes the effects of illness and of mortality. Later, a revised equation included a severity factor (Chiang and Cohen, 1973) and most recently the Index has been expressed in terms of the incidence and duration of illness episodes and the probability of transitions between states (Chiang, 1976). Chen (1983) describes an index based upon the Health Goals Model of Breslow and Somers (1977) which is addressed to the maintenance of specific health goals for specific age groups in the context of doctor-patient care. 'Well' populations are considered to have goals in the area of prevention, while 'sick' populations have theirs in the domain of treatment. 'Sick' and 'well' populations are each divided into ten stages of life from prenatal to old age to give 20 groups. The Index assumes that prevailing medical opinion is the best guide to deciding if certain signs and symptoms warrant medical attention. Thus a need is met if attention is sought and vice versa. The formula incorporates the percentage of people with needs which are met wholly or in part and the index is the geometrical mean of the p. values, i.e. the proportion in each group whose needs are met. This gives a measure of the status of met health needs, not why the needs exist or why they might not be met and is designed mainly for health planners. Its major drawbacks are the availability and collectability of the requisite data and its assumptions about physician-defined needs.

Other single, global indices have been developed. In particular there is interest in 'Quality-adjusted life years' (QALYS) which could be used as units of health benefits and which would be more sensitive than life expectancy, since they would take into account that some interventions may prolong life at the expense of the quality of that life and that some activities may improve quality of life whilst leaving longevity unaffected (Williams, 1983). However, as long ago as 1936 it was remarked, after a review of statistics for indicating population health, that a single index was not heuristic, leading as it does to a serious loss of information (Stouman and Falk, 1936). Nevertheless, refinements of global indices are still being made and their use advocated as the best guide to resource allocation (see, for example, Hurst, 1983). Criticisms of global indices have been dealt with by assuming that a healthy way of life is of equal value to all people, such that aggregation is based upon a universal value. The simplification of

policy options when a 'health' score and a cost
score can be produced giving a ratio of health
points to costs is undoubtedly attractive (Weinstein
and Stason, 1976) but it does seem that we are a
long way from deriving such a health score which
would be appropriate to the particular medical,
social and economic conditions of the industrialised
world.

CHOICE OF A HEALTH INDICATOR

It is clear from the small selection of indicators
reviewed here that the type and form of existing
health measures is very great. Ultimately, the
choice of any one will depend upon the purpose for
which it is to be used; the more specific the
problem, the more specific the indicator will need
to be; the more subtle any presumed changes in
health, the more sensitive the instrument required.
If the need is to evaluate quality of care, clearly
the choice of instrument will be different from a
situation where one is determining priorities for
resource allocation at a population level.
Community surveys may require different instruments
than clinical trials. Indicators may be used to
evaluate hospital or community care, to detect unmet
needs or the presence of disease, to quantify the
impact of illness on everyday life, to predict
utilisation of services, to examine costs and
benefits of particular interventions, to assess
quality of life in chronic disease or to determine
priorities. In general, before deciding on a
particular instrument, for whatever purpose, there
are several issues that will need clarification.

1. What exactly is it that this instrument
   measures? Is it limitation of physical
   function, social disability, emotional
   problems, or the presence of medical
   symptoms?

2. For what populations is the instrument to
   be used? In a sample of a general
   population only about 20 per cent will
   have chronic physical or emotional
   problems, so that a measure based upon
   physical or mental disability or on rather
   severe negative aspects of health will
   tell little about the majority of respondents. On the other hand a sample of
   people with serious health problems may

require a highly specific enquiry.
3. Are the scores expressed in a way which will enable them to be linked easily to other relevant variables?
4. What is the history of the instrument? How have validity and reliability been tested and on what types and numbers of people? How valid and reliable is the measure?
5. On what types of samples has the instrument been standardised? Are the individuals who have been involved in the development and testing of the instrument sufficiently similar to the proposed study population so as not to pose problems of appropriateness? Do norms exist for comparative purposes?
6. If the instrument is to be used for monitoring the effects of a particular intervention, will it measure those aspects of health or disability which are susceptible to change, especially within the time span of the study?
7. How appropriate is the instrument for the proposed population in terms of its administration and response categories? Self report measures may present problems to frail elderly people, those with poor eyesight or arthritic hands and those of poor mental status. Long complex questionnaires are not suitable for ill people and a complicated scoring and computational system may tax the skills of research assistants unused to mathematical techniques.

Where administration of a questionnaire must be by interview, thought must be given to the standardisation of interviewer behaviour, the length of time involved and issues of interviewer/interviewee interaction. If patients are to be observed and rated by an informant, some assessment should be made of the reliability of the information and no instrument should be used without a pilot test on a relevant population

Finally, careful thought should be given to whether administration of a standardised instrument or scale is necessary at all and to what degree it will benefit the respondents. Attempts, for example, to assess quality of life in severely ill patients might well be sensibly founded in a few sympathetic questions to the patient or caretaker, rather than on the presentation of a taxing questionnaire.

REFERENCES

Bergner, M. Bobbitt, R.A. Pollard, W.E. Martin, D.P. and Gilson, B.S. (1976) 'The Sickness Impact Profile: Validation of a Health Status Measure', Med Care, 14, 57-67

Bergner, M. Bobbitt, R.A. Carter, W.B. and Gilson, B.S. (1981) 'The Sickness Impact Profile: Development and Final Revision of a Health Status Measure', Med Care, 19, 787-805

Bradburn, N.M. (1969) The Structure of Psychological Well-Being, Aldine Publishing Co, Chicago

Breslow, L. and Somers, A.R. (1977) 'The Long-term Health Monitoring Program: A Practical Approach to Preventive Medicine', New Eng J Med, 296, 601-608

Brodman, K. Erdman, A.J. and Wolff, H.G. (1960) Cornell Medical Index - Health Questionnaire Manual, Cornell University Medical College, New York

Bush, J.W. (1984) 'General Health Policy Model/ Quality of Well-Being (QWB) Scale' in N.K. Wenger, M.E. Mattson, C.D. Furberg, and J. Elinson (eds.), Assessment of Quality of Life in Clinical Trials of Cardiovascular Therapies Le Jacq Publishing Co, New York, pp. 189-199

Cairl, R.E. Pfeiffer, E. Keller, D.M. Burke, H. and Samis, H.V. (1983) 'An Evaluation of the Reliability and Validity of the Functional Assessment Inventory', J Amer Geriat Soc, 31, 607-612

Chambers, L.W. (1982) The McMaster Health Index Questionnaire (MHIQ) Methodologic Documentation and Report of Second Generation of Investigations, Department of Clinical Epidemiology and Biostatistics, McMaster University, Hamilton, Ontario

Chambers, L.W. MacDonald, L.A. Tugwell, P. Buchanan, W.W. and Kraag, G. (1982) 'The McMaster Health Index Questionnaire as a Measure of Quality of Life for Patients with Rheumatoid Disease', J Rheum, 9, 780-784

Chen, M.K. (1983) 'A Health Needs Index Based on the Health Goals Model', Pub Hlth Reps, 98, 181-184

Chiang, C.L. (1965) An Index of Health: Mathematical Models, Public Health Service Publ. No. 1000, Series 2, No. 5, National Center for Health Statistics, US Government Printing Office, Washington DC

Chiang, C.L. (1976) 'Making Annual Indexes of Health', Hlth Serv Res, 11, 442-451

Chiang, C.L. and Cohen, R.D. (1973) 'How to Measure Health: A Stochastic Model for an Index of Health', Int J Epidemiol, 20, 7-13

Curtis, S. (1983) Intra-urban Variations in Health Health and Health Care: The Comparative Need for Health Care Survey of Tower Hamlets and Redbridge, Vol. 1, Adult Morbidity and Service Use, Queen Mary College, London

Department of Health and Social Security (1976) Sharing Resources in England, Report of the Resource Allocation Working Party, HMSO, London

Dupuy, H.J. (1974) Utility of the National Center for Health Statistics General Well-Being Schedule in the Assessment of Self-Representations of Subjective Well-Being and Distress, National Conference on Evaluation in Alcohol, Drug Abuse and Mental Health Programs, Washington DC

Fillenbaum, G.G. and Smyer, M.A. (1981) 'The Development, Validity and Reliability of the OARS Multidimensional Functional Assessment Questionnaire', J Geront, 36, 428-433

Fries, J.F. Spitz, P.W. and Young, D.Y. (1982) 'The Dimensions of Health Outcome. The Health Assessment Questionnaire: Disability and Pain Scales', J Rheum, 9, 789-793

Goldberg, D.P. (1971) The Detection of Psychiatric Illness by Questionnaire, Oxford University Press, London

Grogono, A.W. and Woodgate, D.J. (1971) 'Index for Measuring Health', Lancet, 2, 1024-1026

Gurland, B.J. Kuriansky, J.B. Sharpe, L. Simon, R. Stiller, P. and Birkett, P. (1977) 'The Comprehensive Assessment and Referral Evaluation (CARE) Rationale, Development and Reliability', Int J Aging and Human Dev, 8, 9-42

Hannay, D. (1978) 'Symptom Prevalence in the Community', J Roy Coll Gen Pract, 28, 492-499

Harris, A.I. (1971) Handicapped and Impaired in Great Britain, HMSO, London

Hurst, J. (1983) 'A Government Economist's Attitudes to the New Measures' in G. Teeling

Smith (ed.), Measuring the Social Benefits of Medicine, Office of Health Economics, London, pp. 139-145

Kaplan, R.M. Bush, J.W. and Berry, C.C. (1976) 'Health Status: Types of Validity and the Index of Well-Being', Hlth Serv Res, 11, 478-507

Katz, S. Ford, A.B. Moskowitz, R.W. Jacobson, B.A. and Jaffe, M.W. (1963), 'The Index of ADL: A Standardised Measure of Biological and Psychological Function', JAMA, 185, 914-919

Katz, S. Ford, A.B. Heiple, K.G. and Newhill, V.A. (1964) Studies of Illness in the Aged: Recovery after Fracture of the Hip', J Geront, 19, 236-242

Katz, S. Ford, A.B. Chinn, A.B. and Newhill, V.A. (1966) 'Prognosis after Strokes: Long Term Course of 159 Patients', Medicine, 45, 236-242

Langner, T.S. (1962) 'A 22-Item Screening Score of Psychiatric Symptoms Indicating Impairment', J Hlth Hum Behav, 3, 269-276

Leavey, R. (1982) Inequalities in Urban Primary Care: Use and Acceptability of GP Services, Department of General Practice, DHSS Research Unit, University of Manchester, Manchester

Martini, C.J.M. Allan, G.J.B. Davison, Jan and Backett, E.M. (1979) 'Health Indexes Sensitive to Medical Care Variation' in J. Elinson and A.E. Seigman (eds.), Socio-medical Health Indicators, Baywood Publishing Co. Inc., New York, pp. 145-164

McDowell, I. and Roberts, J. (1983) 'The Thirty Item Screening Scale: A Survey Measurement of Low-Level Disability', Can J Publ Health, 74, 202-207

Meenan, R.F. Gertman, P.M. and Mason, J.H. (1980) 'Measuring Health Status In Arthritis. The Arthritis Impact Measurement Scales', Arth Rheum, 23, 146-152

Miller, J.E. (1970) 'An Indicator to Aid Management in Assigning Program Priorities', Pub Hlth Reps, 85, 725-729

Office of Population Censuses and Surveys, Social Survey Division (1973) The General Household Survey. Introductory Report, An interdepartmental survey sponsored by the Central Central Statistical Office, HMSO, London

Office of Population Censuses and Surveys, Social Survey Division (1975, 1976, 1977, 1978, 1979, 1980, 1981, 1982) The General Household Survey 1972-1979, HMSO, London

Parkerson, G.R. Gehlbach, S.H. Wagner, E.H. James,

S.A. Clapp, N.E. and Muhlbaier, L.H. (1981) 'The Duke - UNC Health Profile. An Adult Health Status Instrument for Primary Care', Med Care, 19, 806-823

Patrick, D. (1981) 'Standardisation of Comparative Health Status Measures: Using Scales Developed in America in an English-speaking Country' in S. Sudman (ed.), Health Survey Research Methods: Third Biennial Conference, Hyattsville Md. National Center for Health Services Research, PHS Publ. No. 81-3268, pp. 216-220

Patrick, D. Darby, S.C. Green, S. Horton, G. Locker, D. and Wiggins, R.D. (1981) 'Screening for Disability in the Inner City', J Epidemiol Comm Hlth, 35, 65-70

Rosser, R. and Kind, P. (1978) 'A Scale of Valuations of States of Illness: Is There a Social Consensus?', Int J Epidem, 7, 347-357

Rutstein, D.D. Berenberg, W. Chalmers, T.C. Fishman, A.P. Perrin, S. and Zuidema, G.D. (1980) 'Measuring the Quality of Medical Care: Second Revision of Tables of Indexes', New Eng J Med, 302, 1146

Stouman, K. and Falk, I.S. (1936) '"Health Indices": A Study of Objective Indices of Health in Relation to Environment and Sanitation', Bull of the Health Organisation League of Nations, 5, 901-996

Sullivan, D.F. (1966) Conceptual Problems in Developing an Index of Health, U.S. Department of Health Education and Welfare, Publ. No. (HRA) 74-1017, Series 2, No. 5, Washington DC

Sullivan, D.F. (1971) A Single Index of Mortality and Morbidity, HMAHA Health Reports, 347-355, Washington DC

Teresi, J.A. Golden, R. and Gurland, B.J. (1984) 'Concurrent and Predictive Validity of Indicator Scales Developed for the Comprehensive Assessment and Referral Evaluation Interview Schedule', J Geront, 39, 158-165

Ware, J.E. (1976) 'Scales for Measuring General Health Perceptions', Hlth Serv Res, II, 396-415

Weinstein, M.C. and Stason, W.B. (1976) Hypertension: A Policy Perspective, Harvard University Press, Harvard, Mass.

Williams, A. (1983) 'The Economic Role of "Health Indicators"' in G. Teeling-Smith (ed.), Measuring The Social Benefits of Medicine, Office of Health Economics, London, pp. 63-67

Williams, R.G.A. Johnston, M. Willis, L.A. and Bennett, A.E. (1976) 'Disability: A Model and a Measurement Technique', <u>Brit J Prev Soc Med</u>, <u>30</u>, 71-78

Chapter 4.

SELF REPORT AND SUBJECTIVE HEALTH STATUS

The development and use of a health indicator based
upon the perceptions of the general public
inevitably raises issues pertaining to the
reliability of the measurement of subjective
experience. The notion of dualism, i.e. that there
exist separate physical and mental worlds is a very
strong and prevailing one in western culture and the
relationship between 'subject' and 'object' has been
a topic of debate since before the Greco-Roman era.

In general, the common view has been that to
qualify as an object the entity in question must be
antecedent to the experience of it and must be
given, that is, received from the outer world and
not be a mode of reception or something generated by
the perceptual experience (Whitehead, 1964).

Thus we may say that the process of
experiencing is made up of the reception of objects
into the unity that is the process. It follows that
experiences arising within a person are not
'objective' since they 'belong' to the individual
having the experience in a way that objects do not.
Perceptions, since they are not antecedent to
experience, but rather co-terminous and not given
but generated are also, ipso facto, subjective.

This formulation of external and internal
worlds and the relationship between them has led to
much speculation, but little resolution.
Historically, with the exception of the Idealists,
we have been inclined to regard objects as somehow
more real and reliable than experiences, since they
are believed to have an existence independent of the
observer and are, therefore, unchanged (vide
Heisenberg) by being observed and regardless of who
is doing the observing, in a way that perception and
experience are not. Indeed at the very basis of
current methods in Science is the implication that,

61

as far as possible, idiosyncratic impressions should be eliminated by replications and controls which will lead us ever closer to 'objective' truth.

However, as Strasser (1963) has written, 'the object is a discovery made by humans and that objectivity is the result of a certain subjective approach'. Objects may well exist independently of the observer, but 'objectivity', so-called, does not necessarily imply some true and accurate knowledge of the external world but is rather the consequence of a consensus, a sort of subjective collectivism. Therefore, since objectivity is a form of agreement on what entities and events should be regarded as facts, alternative structuring of the objective is always possible.

> ... since we have come to understand that science is not a description of reality but a metaphorical ordering of experience it is not a question of which view is 'true' in some ultimate sense, rather it is a matter of which picture is more useful in guiding human affairs.

(Harman, 1974).

The role of consensus in objectifying the world is well illustrated by the case of professions. One of the defining characteristics of a profession is that it has taken to itself the right to describe the content, methods and forms of its activities in a way which casts the lay person as an outsider. Denied access to the esoteric language, training and appropriate skills and techniques, he or she is constrained to accept the 'objective' opinion of the professional.

Those who make their living as scientists agree to follow a set of rules and procedures commonly agreed to be the 'best' way to discovery of the underlying truth of things. However, as Feyerabend (1975) has pointed out, this represents little more than the acceptance of prevailing ideology. Science is but one of the many forms of thought that have been developed and is not inevitably the best. Indeed both Koestler (1964) and Kuhn (1965) have drawn attention, albeit in very different ways, to the manner in which scientific method and thought is relative to social and ideological trends.

Although Medicine does not lay claim to being a science, the profession has gradually established jurisdiction over matters relating to health, disease, illness, disability and treatment. As such it has prescribed certain 'objective' methods for discerning the presence or absence of disease.

EVALUATING HEALTH STATUS

The evaluation of health status has primarily been made by those methods which are said to yield 'hard data' as opposed, say, to patients' assessments of their conditions, which have generally been considered to be unreliable at best and deliberately intended to mislead at worst.

This professional evaluation by objective means relies heavily on two assumptions; first, that there are disease states which exist independently of medical goals and second that the presence of such states implies an absence of health. Such assumptions are called into question by the fact that the detection of disease and its classification depends upon the stage of medical technology and certain fashions in diagnosis. 'Diseases' tend to differ in degree of status from well-defined, for example, gross congenital malformations, to poorly-defined, for example, alcoholism. Some conditions, detectable only by microtechniques, may be unnoticeable to the patient, who may, therefore, insist on being healthy. Diagnostic categories may be viewed as a 'museum of past and present concepts of disease' (Fabrega, 1973) which are affected by the organisation and state of knowledge of the medical system. Thus 'objective' judgements about disease are relative to time, place and the person making the judgement. Since a verdict of 'healthy' often relates to some 'norm', either statistically in the form of a group average, or by reference to some 'ideal' state there is much room for argument over what exactly is normal or healthy. Since these standards are socially rather than biologically defined, the issue of which or whose definition prevails may often be a question of which group has sufficient power and prestige to enforce its own criteria.

Moreover, the notion that an individual's assessment of his or her own pain and distress is less reliable than professional measures must be set against studies of the accuracy of some 'hard data'. For example, the concordance rate of clinical and pathological diagnoses has been shown to be as low as 45.3 per cent (Heasman and Lipworth, 1966). So-called 'normal' values in biochemistry have been called into question by studies which have documented the arbitrary nature of these values (Bradwell, Carmalt and Whitehead, 1974; Grasbeck and Saris, 1969). The influence of seasonal variations on serum cholestrol readings (Doyle, 1965) and the contingencies underlying conventional judgements of haemoglobin levels (Pryce, 1960) also cast doubt upon the objective nature of some medical opinions.

The problems of establishing a clear demarcation line between 'sick' and 'healthy' have been highlighted by studies of current screening procedures for such disorders as diabetes, hypertension and glaucoma (Cochrane and Holland, 1971). The further one moves from the purely anatomical and physiological the more uncertain do such procedures become. In the field of mental health Szasz and others have drawn attention to the way in which attributions of psychiatric illness are strongly, if not wholly, influenced by a comparison process between the norms and values of the patient and those of the psychiatrist (Szasz, 1971; Goffman, 1961; Scheff, 1961). On the other hand, whilst the presence of physical illness has tended to be deemed to exist if diagnosed by a doctor, psychiatric illness is frequently diagnosed by patients' reports of their mental state.

These differences are, of course, enshrined in the terms signs and symptoms. The former are seen as 'objective' criteria of malfunction (for example, fever, or an elevated white cell count) and the latter are 'subjective' since they are, often, verifiable only by the complainant. When signs and symptoms come into conflict, i.e. the patient complains, but there are no signs of disorder or the doctor finds signs but the patient is asymptomatic, it is, on the whole, the doctor whose opinion carries most weight. At least part of the reluctance to give much weight to patients' reports is related to a fear of malingerers and to the need to maintain professional authority. However, on a more philosophical level it is an issue of the technical competence and criteria of a materialistic science as opposed to the phenomenology of the individual. A technical perspective obviously regards lay persons as incompetent judges of health and disease, but an experiential perspective views individuals as the best judges of their own feelings of well-being or illness. It thus becomes a question of who is judging what. Placing these viewpoints in opposition is neither useful nor necessary. They should both be seen as having merit, complementing each other, or with one perspective being given greater weight depending upon its appropriateness to the circumstances.

Until very recently the province of the evaluation of medical and health care has been exclusively professional. The use of standards and procedures as defined by Medicine and the legal and social responsibility for provision of services has excluded consumer perspectives. Hitherto, the doctor has had the power to make medical norms paramount, so that, for example, radiological evidence and wound healing carry more weight than subjective judgements or a patient's ability to function in a customary manner (Roth, 1963). However, now we are moving into an era when consumers are demanding more participation and control in those areas of medical care where they believe themselves to be the most competent to pronounce. Assessment of the effectiveness of medical procedures has generally focused on quantitative aspects - such as the number of patients treated, time spent in consultations, verification of diagnosis, the technical aspects of surgical operations and outcome measures of chemotherapy, such as five year survival rates. (Allander and Rosenquist, 1975; Gururaj, Russo, Vamedevan, Baltazar, Seth and Pongpavit, 1976; Freeman, 1977; Langman, 1978). However, where physician judgements have been compared to those of patients in relation to outcome, discrepancies have been observed. In a Swedish study there was reported to be only 50 per cent agreement between doctor and patients on whether treatment had been beneficial (Orth-Gomer, Britton and Rehnqvist, 1979) and research on relief from low back pain found little agreement between doctor and patient on whether this had been achieved (Thomas and Lyttle, 1980). An assessment of the results of surgery for peptic ulcer demonstrated disparity between Visick scale scores (based on symptoms and complications of surgery) and patients' experiences. This was most evident in those patients who considered themselves to be fit, following surgery, but who were still having symptoms (Hall, Horrocks, Clamp and DeDombal, 1976).

The work of Cartwright (1964; 1967) has also documented the considerable differences between medical personnel and patients in relation to expectations, values and satisfaction with care. Finlayson and McEwen (1977) showed how even social criteria of recovery traditionally employed by doctors, such as return to work, may be inadequate indicators of restored health since the resumption of employment may only be achieved at the expense of participation in other aspects of daily life such as social and leisure activities. However, there is some evidence to suggest that the gap between patient and medical perceptions is less wide in some specialities. For example, it has been argued that general practitioners are more likely to understand and even share some of the concepts of their patients than are hospital doctors (Helman, 1978).

The increasing proportion of people requiring long term medical and social care has also shifted the emphasis from quantitative, technical, criteria of success towards issues relating to quality of life; a concept which appears quite idiosyncratic and very much related to personal circumstances.

Changes in the structure of the National Health Service in Britain authorised a role for the consumer, notably by the establishment of Community Health Councils in 1974, the setting up of the Hospital Advisory Service and the increased attention paid to hospital complaints procedures (Locker and Dunt, 1978). In the United States, the escalating cost of care, fierce competition for customers and vociferous consumer groups have also led to demands for evaluative procedures which include measures of patient satisfaction and assessment by health care consumers.

However, not all the impetus towards inclusion of patients' views and experience has come from consumers. Indeed Fitzpatrick (1984) has argued that the major pressure has come, rather, from third parties, such as the government, wanting to know more about the value of the services it provides and pays for. Clinicians have also come to recognise the need to incorporate a patient's view of services and outcome (Barsky, 1981).

A major role has been played by research, mainly sociological, which has shown how crucial are subjective elements, such as perceived distress, expectations, social comparison and unmet needs in determining the utilisation of health services. For example, the Health Belief Model, although rather narrow in its assumptions that health-related behaviour is carried out for health reasons, has been successful in the prediction of utilisation of services in both primary care and prevention (Becker, 1974). This model incorporates such phenomenological elements as a subjective state of readiness to act. This in turn is determined by perceived vulnerability plus perceived probability of the seriousness of the condition, in terms of its physical and social consequences; an evaluation of the costs and benefits of seeking care; and some triggering event which will itself be a consequence of a phenomenological event. These variables are also thought to interact with demographic characteristics, such as age, sex and socio-economic status. The Health Belief Model has proved useful in predicting use of immunisation services (Cummings, Jetter, Block and Haefner, 1979), patients' adherence to anti-hypertensive regimes (Kirscht and Rosenstock, 1977) and non-compliance with treatment in end stage renal disease (Hartman and Becker, 1978).

Fabrega (1973) has provided an anthropological approach to health and illness which describes the decision making processes of individuals and which emphasises the subjective nature of judgements made about biological changes, with the 'phenomenologic system' playing a major role in definitions, evaluations and labelling. The general theory of help-seeking for illness developed by Mechanic (1962) also stresses such subjective factors as perceptual salience, perceived seriousness of symptoms, assumptions and understanding, perceived needs and psychological states. A recent review of models of health-related behaviour lists 99 variables found to be influential, at least 42 of which are wholly subjective (Becker and Maiman, 1983). It has been fairly well established that a great deal of utilisation of health services involves symptoms that are widely distributed in the population and which go untreated more frequently than they are treated (White, Williams and Greenberg, 1961). Thus the decision to seek care depends upon a set of contingencies which are involved with the perception of distress.

A major issue in the use of perceived health as an indicator is how far it can be expected that this will relate to 'objective' or physiological status. Does poor subjective health reflect medical problems or is it merely associated with demographic factors which influence social and psychological well-being? It has been argued that belief about health status is an intervening variable between objective health and adoption of the sick role (Maddox, 1964). As a consequence, medical evaluation and self evaluation would be expected to be in agreement except when an individual's estimate of his or her health is erroneous. This incongruity between medical and self assessment is then related to the individual's optimism or pessimism with regard to health. However, this view assumes that medical evaluation is bound to be closer to the actual state of things than self-assessment, a view which, as has been stated earlier, is not necessarily the case. A complicating factor here would obviously be whether the individual has sought medical advice and whether a diagnosis has been received. The first implies that there was some perception of 'dis-ease' and the second, that acceptance or rejection of medical opinion will bear upon the strength of the person's own convictions about the presence of illness and the degree to which the authority of the doctor is recognised as paramount.

PERCEIVED HEALTH AND HEALTH OUTCOME

A number of studies have indicated close relationships between perceived health status and subsequent health outcomes. Over a seven year period substantially increased mortality was observed for people with poor perceived health status even when diagnosed condition and utilisation of health services was controlled for (Mossey and Shapiro, 1982). Similarly, risk of death in a sample of 6928 adults was significantly associated with perceived health when controlling for age, sex, physical health status at the time of rating, health practices, income, education, depression and happiness (Kaplan and Camacho, 1983).

A study of physician utilisation in USA, Yugoslavia and England found perceived morbidity to be the best predictor in each country (Bice and White, 1969). Self-rated health was found to predict morale and return to work after first myocardial infarction (Garrity, 1973), and to be positively associated with relinquishing of the sick role after open heart surgery (Brown and Rawlinson, 1975). Perceived health was also shown to be a predictor of mortality in the Midtown Manhattan study (Singer, Garfinkel, Cohen and Srole, 1976) and has been found to be crucial in adjustment to major illness (National Heart and Lung Institute, 1979).

In a comparison of randomly selected mentally alert elderly persons living in the community with a similar group living in institutions, Fillenbaum (1979) noted that for both male and female community residents, subjective health was consistently and positively related to objective condition. So those who perceived their health status as good and expressed less concern about their health, suffered from fewer illnesses and disabilities and reported fewer health problems. However, this association did not hold for institutionalised subjects and the author suggests that this is because institutions may 'reward' illness behaviour and dependency and also routinely hand out medication so that the inmates begin to consider their health as poor even when they may be judged quite fit medically. It is thus apparent that the context in which self-assessments are made is probably influential in determining their nature. Indeed some writers have suggested that self-reports of health are no more than reflections of morale or self-esteem (Friedman and Martin, 1963; Suchman, Phillips and Streib, 1958). However, this view is contradicted by studies which have found higher agreement between self-ratings of health and ratings of function by physicians, than with measures of morale or self-concept (Tissue, 1972; Palmore and Luikart, 1972).

Relationships between self-reported health status and doctor-assessed health in a sample of 60 year olds followed up over a 15 year period showed a positive and enduring relationship between the two ratings which were stable over time and indicated that self-rating was a better predictor of future physician rating than was the reverse (Maddox and Douglass, 1973). It has been noted frequently that the elderly tend to report better health as they get older and it has been suggested that this is a consequence of the attribution of ailments to ageing rather than declining health (Williamson, Stokde, Gray, Fisher, Smith, McGhee and Stephenson, 1964; Anderson, 1976). However, it may well be that those individuals who do survive into later older age are indeed healthier than younger elderly due to selective mortality. Support for this view comes from a study by Linn and Linn (1980). They measured perceived health on a five point scale ranging from very good to very poor and obtained eight medical indices; impairment assessment and disability rating, number of physician visits, bed days, hospital days, diagnoses, medication and surgical operations. Persons over 75 years reported better health than those aged 65-74, a perception which was supported by the objective measures, with the exception of surgical operations. The authors concluded that self-perceived health may be more useful than age per se as an index of overall health.

In general it appears that the association between subjective and objective health can be specified by careful examination of intervening contextual variables. Obviously self-assessment cannot tell us anything about the incidence and prevalence of specific diseases, but it does provide a useful and accurate guide to general health and tendencies to seek care.

The issue then becomes one of the accurate, valid and reliable assessment of perceived health status via self report. Some self-assessment inventories are no more than lists of clinical conditions which force the lay person to express him or herself in the language of the physician. The idea behind the Nottingham Health Profile was that it should derive its parameters of health status from the perceptions of the lay public, using, initially, 'biographical episodes of illness' (Bennette, 1969) from which could be extracted experiences and modes of expression which would be combined to make a standard indicator of perceived health. Allowing individuals to evaluate their own health status also solves, to a degree, the problems posed by differing definitions of health and illness and has the added advantage of redressing the balance between lay and professional perspectives.

It is neither necessary, nor helpful to see subjective indicators as replacements for the more traditional measures of health status, rather they may be regarded as providing enlightenment, by means of which patterns of thinking about social realities can be rearranged. Data concerned with how people feel in a given set of circumstances can be expressed in a standard manner and can enrich information about how long they live or of what malady they die. Given a broader definition of science which can encompass 'soft' as well as 'hard' data, there is no reason why systems which include subjective information should not be capable of intellectual refinement so that they become amenable to quantification. In this manner important aspects of health-related experience can be tested for validity and reliability and can be used to assess and compare levels of health status.

REFERENCES

Allander, E. and Rosenquist, U. (1975) 'The Diagnostic Process in Outpatient Endocrine Care with Special Reference to Screening. Further

Study of Diagnostic Patterns, their Changes, Total and Diagnosis-Specific Resource Consumption', Scand J Soc Med, 3, 117-121

Barsky, A.J. (1981) 'Hidden Reasons some Patients Visit Doctors', Anns Int Med, 94, 492-498

Becker, M.H. (ed.), (1974) 'The Health Belief Model and Personal Health Behaviour', Health Ed Monog, 2, 324-508

Becker, M. and Maiman, Lois A. (1983) 'Models of Health Related Behaviour' in D. Mechanic (ed.), Handbook of Health, Health Care and the Health Professions, The Free Press, New York, pp. 539-568

Bennette, G. (1969) 'Psychic and Cellular Aspects of Isolation; Identity Impairment in Cancer : a Dialiectic of Alienation', Anns NY Acad Sci, 164, 352-363

Bice, T.W. and Camacho, T. (1983) 'Perceived Health and Mortality: a nine year follow up of the Human Population Laboratory Cohort', Amer J Epidem, 117, 292-298

Bradwell, A.R. Carmalt, M.H.B. and Whitehead, T.P. (1974) 'Explaining the Unexpected Abnormal Results of Biochemical Profile Investigations', Lancet, 2, 1071-1074

Brown, J.S. and Rawlinson, M. (1975) 'Relinquishing the Sick Role Following Open Heart Surgery', J Hlth Soc Behav, 16, 12-27

Cartwright, A. (1967) Patients and their Doctors, Routledge and Kegan Paul, London.

Cartwright, A. (1964) Human Relations and Hospital Care, Routledge and Kegan Paul, London.

Cochrane, A.L. and Holland, W.W. (1971) 'Validation of Screening Procedures', BMJ, 27, 3-8

Cummings, K.M. Jetter, R.P.T. Brock, B.M. and Haefner, D.P. (1979) 'Psychosocial Determinants of Immunisation Behaviour in a Swine Influenza Campaign', Med Care, 17, 639-649

Doule, J.T. (1965) 'Seasonal Variation in Serum Cholesterol Concentration', J Chron Dis, 18, 657-664

Fabrega, H. Jr. (1973) 'Towards a Model of Illness Behaviour', Med Care, 11, 470-484

Feyerabend, P. (1975) Against Method, Verso, London

Fillenbaum, G.G.' Social Context and Self-Assessments of Health Among the Elderly', J Hlth Soc Behav, 20, 45-51

Finlayson, A. and McEwen, J. (1977) Coronary Heart Disease and Patterns of Living, Croom Helm, London

Fitzpatrick, R. (1984) 'Satisfaction with Health

Care' in R. Fitzpatrick, J. Hinton, S. Newman, G. Scrambler, and J. Thompson, The Experience of Illness, Tavistock, London, pp. 154-175

Freeman, M.A.R. (1977) 'Replacement of the Severely Damaged Arthritic Knee by the ICLH (Freeman-Swanson) Arthroplasty', J Bone Joint Surg, 59B, 64-68

Friedman, H.J. and Martin H.W. (1963) 'A Comparison of Self and Physician Health Ratings in an Older Population', J Hlth Soc Behav, 4, 179-183

Garrity, T.F. (1973) 'Vocational Adjustment after First Myocardial Infarction: a Comparative Assessment of Several Variables Suggested in the Literature', Soc Sci Med, 7, 705-717

Goffman, E. (1961) Asylums: Essays on the Social Situation of Mental Patients and Other Inmates, Anchor Books, Garden City

Grasbeck, R. and Saris, N.E. (1969) 'Establishment and Use of Normal Values', Scand J Clin Lab Invest, Suppl, 110, 62-63

Gururaj, V.J. Russo, R.M. Vamedevan, N. Baltazar, O.Z. Seth, K.A. and Pongpavit, C. (1976) 'Patient Flow Analysis in a Municipal Hospital Outpatient Department', NY State J Med, 76, 544-549

Hall, R. Horrocks, J.C. Clamp, S.E. and DeDombal, F.T. (1976) 'Observer Variation in Assessment of Results of Surgery for Peptic Ulceration', B Med J, 1, 814-816

Harman, W. (1974) 'The New Copernican Revolution' Unpublished, Quoted in 'Can Consciousness Make a Difference?', in P. Lee, R.E. Ornstein, D. Gallin, A. Deikman and C.T. Tart (eds.), Symposium on Consciousness, American Association for the Advancement of Science, Viking Press, New York, p. 2

Hartman, P.E. and Becker, M.H. (1978) Non-compliance with Prescribed Regimen Among Chronic Haemodialysis Patients: a Method of Prediction and Educational Diagnosis', Dialysis and Transplantation, 7, 978-989

Heasman, M.A. and Lipworth, L. (1966) 'Accuracy of Certification of Cause of Death', Studies on Medical and Population Subjects, No. 20, General Register Office, HMSO, London

Helman, C.G. (1978) 'Feed a Cold, Starve a Fever - Folk Models of Infection in an English Suburban Community', Cult Med and Psychiat, 2, 107-137

Kaplan, G.A. and Camacho, T. (1983) 'Perceived Health and Mortality : a Nine Year Follow Up of the Human Population Laboratory Cohort', Amer J

Epidem, 117, 292-298

Kirscht, J.P. and Rosenstock, I.M. (1977) 'Patient Adherence to Antihypertensive Medical Regimens', J Comm Hlth, 3, 115-124

Koestler, A. (1964) The Sleepwalkers, Penguin Books, Harmondsworth

Kuhn, T. (1965) The Structure of Scientific Revolutions, University of Chicago Press, Chicago

Langman, M.J. (1978) 'Treatment Trials and Their Design', Clin Gastroenterol, 7, 583-587

Linn, G.S. and Linn, Margaret W. (1980) 'Objective and Self-Assessed Health in the Old and Very Old', Soc Sci Med, 14A, 311-315

Locker, D. and Dunt, D. (1978) 'Theoretical and Methodological Issues in Sociological Studies of Consumer Satisfaction with Medical Care', Soc Sci Med, 12, 283-292

Maddox, G.L. and Douglass, E. (1973) 'Self-Assessment of Health: a Longitudinal Study of Elderly Subjects', J Hlth Soc Behav, 14, 87-93

Maddox, G.L. (1964) 'Self-Assessment of Health Status: a Longitudinal Study of Selected Elderly Subjects', J Chron Dis, 17, 449-460

Mechanic, D. (1962) 'The Concept of Illness Behaviour', J Chron Dis, 15, 189-194

Mossey, J.M. and Shapiro, E. (1982) 'Self-Rated Health: a Predictor of Mortality among the Elderly', Amer J Pub Hlth, 72, 800-808

National Heart and Lung Institute (1976) 'Report of a Task Group on Cardiac Rehabilitation' in Proceedings of the Heart and Lung Institute Working Conference on Health Behaviour, Department of Health, Education and Welfare, Bethesda, Maryland

Orth-Gomer, K. Britton, M. and Rehnqvist, N. (1979) 'Quality of Care in an Outpatient Department: the Patients' View', Soc Sci Med, 13A, 347-351

Palmore, E. and Luikart, C. (1972) 'Health and Social Factors Related to Life Satisfaction', J Hlth Soc Behav, 13, 68-72

Pryce, J.D. (1960) 'Level of Haemoglobin in Whole Blood and Red Blood Cells and Proposed Convention for Defining Normality', Lancet, 2, 333

Roth, J.A. (1963) Timetables, Bobbs Merrill, Indianopolis

Scheff, T. (1961) Becoming Mentally Ill, Aldine, Chicago

Singer, E. Garfinkel, R. Cohen, S.M. and Srole, L. (1976) 'Mortality and Mental Health: Evidence from the Middtown Manhattan Re-Study', Soc Sci Med, 10, 517-521

Strasser, S. (1963) Phenomenology and the Human Sciences, Duquesne University Press, Pittsburgh, p. 60

Suchman, E.A. Phillips, B.S. and Streib, G.F. (1958) 'An Analysis of the Validity of Health Questionnaires', Social Forces, 36, 232-246

Szasz, T. (1971) The Manufacture of Madness, Routledge and Kegan Paul, London

Thomas, M.R. and Lyttle, D. (1980) 'Patient Expectations about Success of Treatment and Reported Relief from Low Back Pain', J Psychom Res, 24, 297-301

Tissue, T. (1972) 'Another Look at Self-Rated Health and the Elderly', J Geront, 27, 91-94

White, K.L. Williams, T.F. and Greenberg, B.G. (1981) 'The Ecology of Medical Care', New Eng J Med, 265, 885-892

Whitehead, A.M. (1964) Adventures of Ideas, Cambridge, University Press, Cambridge

Williamson, J. Stokde, I.J. Gray, S. Fisher, M. Smith, A. McGhee, A. and Stephenson, E. (1964) 'Old People at Home and Their Unreported Needs', Lancet, 1, 1117-1120

Chapter 5.

DEVELOPING AN INDICATOR OF PERCEIVED HEALTH

The last chapter argued that patients' perceptions of their own health are as good as, if not sometimes better than, clinical predictions of ill heath and mortality. Simply providing people with lists of clinical conditions is no short cut to measuring perceived health status, as they force lay subjects to think and to express their problems in the language of the physician. The development of measures in which the parameters of health status are derived from the perceptions of lay people using the language of illness to describe experiences of ill health present modes of expression which are readily understood by those who complete the finished instrument. Whatever the form of a perceived health measure, it is essential that the health statements or items included in it are derived from a lay population. Constructing instruments in this way avoids the need to define health precisely or in ways that have little meaning for non-clinicians.

Prior to the construction of a measure of perceived health a number of decisions have to be made. The major of these are; how items should be derived for inclusion in the instrument, which methods of scaling to choose, and whether or not all items should be allocated equal importance or whether they should be weighted to reflect relative severity.

The most important point to note is that the concern is with 'perceptions' of health rather than some objective fact which is independent of the individual's experience. Blood pressure can be objectively measured but the way in which a low or high blood pressure is experienced is a perception, and that perception will vary from individual to individual. Similarly, people will differ in their sensitivity to anxiety or changes in mood.

SELECTING ITEMS FOR INCLUSION IN A PERCEIVED HEALTH MEASURE

The items included in an instrument designed to measure perceived health will generally take the form of statements about health. Four main methods of generating items are available: writing one's own, gathering statements from the literature, asking experts to provide relevant items or collecting statements from lay patients and/or non-patients. The method selected will largely be governed by the purpose of the measure.

In traditional psychological measurement, items or statements have generally been written by the person developing the measure. A large pool of statements is produced and each is then tested out in a number of ways, checking for such requisites as lack of ambiguity, meaningfulness, relevance, internal consistency and an ability to discriminate between subjects with differing attitudes. Such an approach may well provide a test which is psychometrically good but which may reflect the understanding and attitude of the test-constructor (although there are ways of overcoming such problems).

Items can also be selected from literature reviews (which will probably reflect expert opinion) or from content analysis of pilot questions which have allowed open-ended responses. In the latter case, items generated should certainly be of relevance to future samples completing the measure but the method is limited by the size of the initial sample employed and the individual's perceptions and experiences of the topic area.

Using experts to generate items has its own problems, especially in the field of perceived health. There is a danger that the final set of statements will reflect objective assessments of health and consequently be similar to existing objective measures.

Probably the most valid way of selecting items for a measure of perceived health is to approach lay people and ask them about the kind of health problems they have experienced. This approach has a number of advantages. The test developer is less likely to impose his or her own values on the pool of items, the statements can be written in the same or similar way to that in which they were generated,

they will reflect the issues and problems which are
of relevance to the people who will be subsequently
completing the test and symptoms can be described in
the way in which they are experienced by 'non-
experts'.

The choice of method for selecting items will
also depend on the type of scaling used. For
example, when constructing Guttman-type items (see
below) it will probably be necessary for the test
constructor or experts to select the statements in
order that logical grades of problems can be listed.

SELECTION OF METHOD OF SCALING

Scaling is necessary where answers given by a
respondent need to be combined to give a measurement
of, for example, intensity or extremity of an
attitude, or more relevantly the severity of a
health problem. If it is assumed that pain problems
can be measured on a scale from no pain through to,
say, severe chronic pain, then some form of scaling
is required to place an individual on this
continuum. The simplest form of scaling would be to
present the subject with a line labelled 'no pain'
at one end and 'severe chronic pain' at the other
and ask him or her to mark whereabouts on that line
they would judge their pain to be. Of course, this
would be a very crude measure and relatively
difficult for the respondent to understand and carry
out. Generally, a more accurate method would
involve asking a number of questions about pain and
then adding the answers together in some way - by
some form of scaling.

The three most widely used scaling methods are
the method of paired comparisons, rank order methods
and rating scales.

The method of paired comparisons is generally
used at the stage of text development and is
designed to simplify the job of people who are
rating items on some criterion, such as the severity
of health problems. Instead of presenting each
subject with five statements about pain and asking
him or her to put them in order of severity, the
task can be simplified by presenting two at a time.
For five pain statements (a,b,c,d and e) ten pairs
of statements can be constructed and so ten
judgements would be required. If, say, 50 people
are asked to make these ten judgements then the five
pain statements can be ordered in terms of severity.
For example, if statement 'a' is judged more severe

than statement 'b' forty times and 'b' rated more severe than 'a' ten times, then the consensus view is that 'a' represents a more severe pain problem. However, it will often be the case that two or more statements are not so clearly differentiated by people making the judgements. For example, it is possible that 25 people might judge statement 'd' more severe than statement 'e' and 25 judge 'e' more severe than 'd'. As will be shown later, this method of scaling allows weights to be calculated for each statement representing its severity as judged by the respondents. In this case 'b' would clearly have a higher weighting than 'a' (indicating greater severity) while 'd' and 'e' would have similar weights attached. Interested readers should consult Thurstone (1927a and 1927b) for an exhaustive discussion of paired comparison techniques.

Rank ordering is commonly used as a scaling technique, mainly because of the ease of computation of scores. If we consider the five pain statements again, they would be presented together to the respondent who would be required to place them in order of severity from one to five. It can be seen that the method is very similar to that of paired comparisons in that each statement can be compared with all the others, albeit simultaneously. However, paired comparisons allow deviations from a strict rank order, while rank ordering forces a judge to display a certain internal consistency which could be artificial. For example, where a judge considers statements A, B and C to be of about the same severity, it is possible to obtain judgements such as A>B, B>C, C>A. The apparent lack of logic in such judgements is likely to be an indication of equivalence which is not possible where A, B and C must be placed in rank order.

It is possible to convert rank order judgements into paired comparisons and derive scale values in the ways suggested by Thurstone. Thus if five statements are ordered : A, B, D, E, C, then the following ten comparative judgements result : A>B, A>D, A>E, A>C, B>D, B>E, B>C, D>E, D>C, E>C.

In terms of economy of time the ranking method is superior to that of paired comparisons. Ranking 20 statements is clearly quicker than making 190 paired comparison judgements (190 being the number of possible pairings of 20 statements). Barratt (1914) showed that obtained scale values from both methods are equally valid. However, one must question an individual's ability and/or motivation to rank order, for example, 20 different statements about pain or social isolation in terms of severity. Furthermore, techniques do exist for reducing the number of paired comparison judgements which have to be made in order to determine scale values (Torgerson, 1958). In the case of rating jokes, Conklin and Sutherland (1923) found rating scale methods superior to the method of ranking.

Rating scales are probably the most widely used method of measuring attitudes and personality traits and can readily be used for measuring perceived health. The method assumes that a response can be made at some point on a continuum between two extremes. An extreme example would be a rating of consciousness from coma through to full alertness. In the case of the semantic differential (Osgood, Suci and Tannenbaum, 1957) a straight line is anchored at each end by an adjective describing one end of a semantic continuum. The subject is required to rate the concept by putting a mark on the line where he feels that concept lies. For example, a respondent may be asked to rate his or her sleep on a continuum from satisfying to dissatisfying. In other rating scales, the responses may be very clearly defined: for example, 'how often do you have problems getting to sleep?' may be followed by responses such as : every night, most nights, sometimes, rarely, never - with the respondent required to indicate one response only.

One major decision has to be made when developing a rating scale - the number of scale divisions to use. Clearly, too few divisions will provide a rather coarse measure - possibly little more useful than the simple categorial choice of yes/no or healthy/unhealthy. On the other hand, too many divisions may be beyond the subject's ability to discriminate. The decision is largely empirical depending on the sample size, the nature of the factors being rated and the ability and motivation of raters to discriminate. Conklin (1923) used 23,000 untrained subjects to determine the maximum number of response categories that should be used. He concluded that the maximum should be five for a single scale and nine for a double scale. A single scale is one which extends from zero to a maximum, while a double scale extends through zero from opposite extremes of the continuum, for example, perfect health through to severe health problems. However, rating scales predominantly employ five or seven response categories.

A problem with rating scales is the subject's tendency to avoid the extreme points of the continuum and to check the central point or one close to it. Sometimes an even number of points is selected to force a rater to avoid the central point.

The method of rating scales has certain advantages over paired comparisons and the methods of rank order. Ratings take less time, are generally more interesting to the raters, have a wider range of applications, and can be used with a large number of stimuli or statements about health.

Scale values can be built into a rating scale and a zero point identified. However, these values are generally arbitrarily defined. For example, the responses and associated scale values for the question 'how would you rate your present health compared with how it was six months ago?' might be:

Much better	+ 2
Slightly better	+ 1
About the same	0
Slightly worse	- 1
Much worse	- 2

The scale values assume that the difference between 'about the same' and 'slightly worse' is the same as that between 'much better' and 'slightly better'.

However, this apparently attractive technique is frequently used directly for obtaining indices of various kinds. In contrast, paired comparisons and rank ordering are often used as stages in the development of indices. The development of measures from scaling methods is discussed in the following section.

DEVELOPING INDICES FROM SCALING METHODS

A measure of perceived health will consist of a number of items or statements describing health problems. The person completing the questionnaire will be required to select one response from a number of alternatives or to say whether or not a problem applies. More complex measures do exist but in principle it is better to make the task simple for the respondent.

It may also be desirable to allocate a weight to each item or statement, representing its importance or severity in relation to the other statements. As noted previously, rating scales have built in weights but more complex weighting procedures are necessary when other scaling methods are used.

The weights developed for these other methods are determined by the people who make the initial judgements; in the case of the paired comparisons by the people who initially decide between each pair of items. Thus the weights applied to sleep problems might be expected to differ if the initial judgements were made by doctors, depressed subjects or a relatively healthy lay group. The decision as to who should make the judgement will be determined by the nature of the concept being investigated. If one wished to determine an 'objective' measure of the severity of a variety of sleep problems, one might select a group of doctors to make the initial judgements. However, if one wished to find out how lay people rate the relative severity of the problems, a sample of judges with a history of sleep problems might well be selected. In other situations the selection of judges may be more difficult. If one wished to rate, say, the prestige of occupations, expertness probably has little meaning (although such judgements were made in developing the Registrar General's social classifications, a major variable employed in many surveys of health - particularly in relation to social inequalities).

The method of developing weights from paired comparisons has been touched on briefly. The weights are calculated by considering the proportion of times each statement is judged to be more severe than each of the other statements. An example of the method of deriving weights is described in detail below. Once each statement has been given a weight the total list of statements is presented to a respondent. For each item he or she affirms as true or applicable, that weighted score is achieved. For example, in a scale containing several statements describing health problems, the respondent will obtain a weighted score for each one that applies. The weights for all affirmed items are then added to provide the index of sleep problems. Thus in its final form, the relatively cumbersome and time consuming method of paired comparisons is reduced to a simple checklist.

Thurstone-type scales are a sophisticated form of rating scale (Thurstone, 1959). A large number of statements are derived from various sources; publications, experts, patients, etc. and these are typed on to cards and sorted into eleven piles ranging, say, from minor health problems up to very severe health problems. The scale value for each statement is that of the pile in which the median card with that statement on, is placed. For example, if there are 51 judges assessing the severity of the statement 'I have trouble waking up in the mornings' into eleven piles, eight may place it in pile number 3, ten in number 4, fifteen in number 5, twelve in number 6, and six in the seventh pile. The median (or middle value) is pile number 5 and this would be the scale value given to the statement. Statements which are widely spread across the piles are discarded as are those shown to be irrelevant or ambiguous. The final scale will consist of statements which are unambiguous, relevant and evenly distributed across the range of scale values.

When completing a Thurstone-type scale, the subject marks all statements with which he or she agrees or which apply and the score is the median scale value of the statements which have been endorsed.

The Guttman scalogram technique has some properties in common with Thurstone scaling but is claimed to be totally unidimensional, i.e. measuring one concept only. Stouffer, quoted in Goode and Hatt (1952), refers to Guttman's work on scale analysis as follows:

> He (Guttman) considered an area scalable if responses to a set of items in that area arranged themselves in certain specified ways. In particular it must be possible to order the items such that, ideally, persons who answer a given question favourably all have higher ranks than persons who answer the same question unfavourably. From a respondent's rank or scale score we know exactly which items he endorsed. Thus we can say that the response to any item, provides a definition of the respondent's attitude.

The quality of being able to reproduce the responses to each item, knowing only the total score, is called reproducibility — one of the tests of whether a set of items constitutes a Guttman scale.

A simplistic set of items could be:

1. Do you weigh over 90 kilograms?
2. Do you weigh between 80 and 89 kilograms?
3. Do you weigh between 70 and 79 kilograms?

4.   Do you weigh below 70 kilograms?

Clearly only one concept is being measured and affirming 2 implies a weight greater than those defined in 3 and 4 but less than that defined in 1.
The Beck Depression Inventory (Beck, Mendleson and Erbaugh, 1961) consists of items in a Guttman scale form. For example:

1.   I do not feel sad.
2.   I feel blue or sad.

1.   I am blue or sad all the time and I can't snap out of it.
2.   I am so sad or unhappy that it is very painful.
3.   I am so sad or unhappy that I can't stand it.

Although respondents are asked to tick the statement which most nearly applies to them, it is possible that more than one could apply. The following set of items in the inventory do appear to form a suitable Guttman scale:

I haven't lost much weight, if any, lately
I have lost more than 5 pounds
I have lost more than 10 pounds
I have lost more than 15 pounds

although checking the last item makes the second and third true but not the first. Finally the set of items:

I am no more irritated now than I ever am
I get annoyed or irritated more easily than I used to
I feel irritated all the time
I don't get irritated at all at things that used to irritate me

seems to be totally unscaled.

Rating scales are superior in the ease with which they allow the construction of indices. The simplest (and perhaps one of the most useful) indicators of perceived health is the item 'How would you rate your present health?' An appropriate response scale might be (1) excellent, (2) good, (3) fair, (4) poor, (5) very poor. The respondent's perceived health index will then be 1, 2, 3, 4, or

5. However, more detailed indices can be constructed by increasing the number of items to, say, 20, allowing scores to range from 20 to 100. It should be noted that any score other than 20 or 100 could be obtained in a number of different ways. This presents no problem where all 20 items are measuring the same concept and are of equal importance. However, this is most unlikely to be the case. Consider a 20-item measure of perceived health which covered physical, psychological and social problems. Three individuals may obtain the score of 60 but each may be scoring highly in a different domain, with relatively low scores in the other two. In such a situation the overall score or index alone does not suggest the nature of the perceived health problems.

The most commonly used rating scale technique follows the approach of Likert (1932). This procedure does not require the classification of items by a group of judges (as in Thurstone scaling) but relies on the responses of subjects during the development of the test. A graded response is required to each statement, commonly these are: strongly agree, agree, undecided, disagree, and strongly disagree. Statements are generally clearly favourable or unfavourable, especially where attitudes are being measured.

Perhaps the most widely used Likert-type scale of perceived health is the General Health Questionnaire (GHQ) developed by Goldberg (1972). Although this measure is called a 'general health questionnaire' it is a self-administered screening test designed to detect non-psychotic psychiatric disorder.

Respondents are asked to compare themselves in the past few weeks (months or some other specified time period) with how they usually feel. Occasionally respondents are simply asked to indicate how they have been feeling recently. The items cover a number of separate domains including sleep, concentration, mood and stress. The following two items show that the response scales vary:

1. Lost much sleep over worry; not at all, no more than usual, rather more than usual, much more than usual.
2. Been able to face up to your problem; more so than usual, same as usual, less able than usual, much less able.

In the case of (1) a respondent can show only
health problems, while in (2) he or she can indicate
improved perceived health. Despite this and the
range of domains, the GHQ is usually scored 0, 1, 2
or 3 for each item, with all items summed to give a
total score. Goldberg recommends that Likert-type
scoring should not be used and that a simple 0 or 1
score should be assigned to each response: zero to
the first two categories and one where one of the
two extreme responses has been checked. Where a
certain proportion of statements have received a
score of one (usually 20 per cent) the respondent is
considered to be a 'case'. The statements are not
weighted for severity.

In practice, the measure appears to work quite
well in reflecting changes in perceived health
following changes in status, for example, when
becoming unemployed or when regaining employment.
However, a problem with the GHQ is the nature
of the instructions and the response scales.
Theoretically, an individual with a chronic but
stable non-psychotic psychiatric disorder should
obtain a low score. In practice, respondents appear
to disregard the instructions and indicate their
distress by treating the response scales as ranging
from no problem to a severe problem.

The foregoing discussion has been concerned
with the ways in which scaling techniques can and
have been used to design measures of perceived
health. Measures based on other models could also be
used, for example: economic models, disabilty
indices and symptom/function indices, as described
in chapter 3. However, such models are less well
supported theoretically and sometime lead to the
development of indicators which are much more
demanding of the respondents.

The next section of this chapter describes the
development of the Nottingham Health Profile and
illustrates a number of the themes which have been
discussed so far.

THE DEVELOPMENT OF THE NOTTINGHAM HEALTH PROFILE

In 1975 a research team in the Department of
Community Health at the University of Nottingham
began work on a 'quality of life' measure intended
to act as an indicator describing the typical
effects of ill health: physical, social and
emotional.

Such an instrument was required to aid

decision-making for health care and to help in determining more accurately the needs and problems of the community. The reason for collecting health information is to assist in management of the services needed by the population. Consequently patients'subjective needs are equally as important as their objective needs.

Specifically, this measure of the quality of life was intended to:

1. Provide some assessment of a person's need for care which was not based upon purely medical criteria.
2. Enable the subsequent evaluation of care provided for persons in need.
3. Make a start on the development of an indicator which could be used for the survey of population health status.

The rationale for such a measure has been discussed at some length in the first four chapters of this book.

The research team began by interviewing 768 patients with a variety of acute and chronic ailments. These interviews produced 2,200 statements describing the effects of ill health. The statements were grouped according to the function described; sleeping, eating, mobility, social life, emotional reactions and so on. The wording of each statement was scrutinised for redundancy, ambiguity, understandability, clarity, ease of reading, esoteric expressions and reading age required (using the Dale 3000 word list). Following this procedure 138 statements remained.

Combinations of these statements were tested out in a number of studies between 1976 and 1978 to further reduce and refine the number of statements.

Scores on the questionnaires were related to medical information and independent assessments of patients' well-being, and it was found that the items were reliable and valid in distinguishing between different degrees of disability. The items were also able to distinguish between physical and mental disorders (Martini and McDowell, 1976 and 1977; McDowell and Martini, 1976; McDowell, Martini and Waugh, 1978).

Following these studies, 82 statements remained which had shown their value in reflecting subjective health states and which had a high degree of salience. These statements provided a measure of perceived disability and handicap. The work of

Martini and McDowell had shown than an index of subjective well-being was a feasible proposition in terms of acceptability and potential sensitivity. Therefore, it was decided that the original objective should be expanded, in order to test the use of the index as an evaluative tool and as an instrument for population survey. This change required a somewhat different approach to that previously adopted.

The ultimate objective of this new approach was to produce a valid and reliable indicator of perceived health status for use on populations, which could be included as part of a comprehensive health survey. It was envisaged that the indicator would contribute to:

1. The identification of groups in need of care.
2. The development of social policy, by helping to determine the allocation of resources.
3. Mass aspects of the evaluation of health and social services.
4. The identification of consumer concerns.
5. The theoretical understanding of differential responses to comparable pathologies.

Work started on this second stage of the development of the NHP in 1978.

A closer look was taken at the remaining statements and they were retested and analysed using the following criteria for selection: there should be no negative expressions, statements should be easy to understand, unambiguous and easy to answer preferably by 'yes' or 'no'. Once an item had satisfied these criteria it was tested out on a sample of patients and non-patients for clarity, consensus of meaning and ease of answering. Those statements which passed the tests were retained. This left a final pool of 38 statements which fell into six sections; physical mobility, pain, sleep, social isolation, emotional reactions and energy level.

Weighting the Statements
Two different factors influenced the way in which the measure was to be scored. First, it was necessary to treat the sections separately as the features of pain, social isolation and so on, are

qualitatively distinct and made up of different facets without common denominators. It would be meaningless simply to add up the number of affirmative responses out of the 38 possible. Thus the measure changed from being an index to a profile in which a different score is obtained for each section. While this made scoring more complex, it allowed more information to be used and scores to be expressed in the form of visual analogues.

The second factor influencing scoring was that of the relative severity of items within the sections. For example, the presence of constant pain might well be considered a more severe problem than having pain when walking. As has been discussed earlier in the chapter, it is common practice to weight items in order to determine their relative importance and such weightings are dependent upon scale values developed from some form of scaling.

The method of scaling to be used was partly influenced by the way in which statements had been collected; from lay respondents. Guttman scaling was inappropriate because items were not clearly graded (see above) and because it was decided that the weightings should be determined by lay respondents, in order to maintain the 'subjective' nature of the measure. Rank ordering was considered too complex and time consuming for untrained respondents. Likert-type scaling was thought to be inappropriate as all statements referred to relatively severe health problems and would lead to highly skewed ratings and little discrimination between items.

The most appropriate technique for weighting, appeared to be that provided by Thurstone's Method of Paired Comparisons, which allowed empirical judgements based on perceived differences to be made.

Subjects drawn from patient and non-patient groups were asked to judge each statement in a section against every other statement in that section, in terms of which condition or situation they considered to be worse. Statements were paired at random, with the order of presentation reversed for half the interviews. In all, 1,200 interviews were carried out, 200 on each of the sections. The age range of respondents was between 18 and 75 with slightly more females than males interviewed.

The method by which weights were derived are reported in detail in McKenna, Hunt and McEwen (1981) but are summarised here. There are two stages in the development of weights. First, it is necessary to determine the scale values of each statement and second, from the scale values to calculate the actual weights. These processes can best be shown by example:

Let us assume that 200 people were asked to rate the relative seriousness of three statements: A, B and C, which were presented two at a time. Table 5.1 shows the type of frequency of response which may result.

The table shows that statement A was rated more severe than statement B by 160 people and more severe than statement C by 150 people. In contrast, 40 people rated statement B more severe than statement A and 50 people rated statement C more severe than statement A. Statement B was also rated more severe than statement C by a majority of the subjects.

Table 5.1 is known as the frequency of response matrix or Matrix F. Table 5.2 shows the proportion matrix or Matrix P.

Table 5.1: Matrix F - Frequency Matrix showing the Number of Times Each Statement was judged More Severe than the Other Two (hypothetical data)			
	Statement Rated More Severe		
	A	B	C
Statement Rated Less Severe A	-	40	50
B	160	-	60
C	150	140	-

The matrix is constructed from Matrix F. The values in the cells are the proportion of times each statement was judged a greater problem than the others. The diagonal cells can be left blank or the value 0.5 can be entered, as it assumed that if respondents were required to compare a statement

with itself the first and second item would be
selected an equal number of times.
    From Matrix P, Matrix X (Table 5.3) - the basic
transformation matrix - is constructed. The cell
values are the unit normal deviates corresponding to

Table 5.2: Matrix P - Proportion Matrix showing the
Proportion of Times Each Statement was judged more
severe than the other two (hypothetical data)

	A	B	C
A	0.50	0.20	0.25
B	0.80	0.50	0.30
C	0.75	0.70	0.50

the proportions.   The values are positive when the
proportion is greaterthan 0.5, and negative when the
proportion is less than 0.5.
    It is not necessary to be conversant with 'unit
normal deviates'.   These values are determined by
referring to the table in a basic statistics book
which gives the areas under the normal curve.   The
proportion value in the body of the table is found
and the corresponding 'z' value read off.   It is
important to include the minus sign if the
proportion is below 0.5.
    Mosteller (1951) and Horst (1941) have shown
that the usual procedure for obtaining estimates of
scale values is a least-square solution.   A
derivation following Mosteller's treatment is given
by Torgeson (op cit).   In practice the scale values
are calculated by summing and averaging the normal
deviate values for each statement.   These
calculations are shown in Table 5.3.
    The scale values are located on the severity
continuum with respect to each other only (and they
total zero).   Torgeson (op cit), when suggesting how
to derive weightings from scale values, argues that
a constant should be added to each scale value in
order that a zero point can be derived.   This leaves

the problem of deciding which constant to add. For example, adding 2 to each value would influence the relative position of each value differently from an addition of 10 to each. McKenna, Hunt and McEwen (op cit) show that a rational zero point can be established by a regression technique. For the present example the zero point would be at $X = -1.335$. The constant 1.335 can then be added to

Table 5.3: Matrix X - Unit Normal Deviates of the Proportions given in Table 5.2

	A	B	C
A	0.00	-0.84	-0.67
B	0.84	0.00	-0.52
C	0.67	0.52	0.00
Sum	1.51	-0.32	-1.19
Mean (Scale Values)	0.503	-0.107	-0.397

each scale value giving: A(Wa) = 1.84, B(Wb) = 1.23, C(Wc) = 0.94 (that is, the distance of each item item from the rational zero).

For the Nottingham Profile it was decided that all sections should allow scores to range from zero (no problems) to 100 (where all problems in the section are affirmed). The weights can be adjusted to fit this requirement by multiplying each by 100/(Wa + Wb + Wc) = 25.03. This gives the final weights:

```
A = 45.93
B = 30.66
C = 23.40
```

Calculations will show that the relative

distance between items is the same for the final weights as for the original scale values.

When scoring the Profile by computer, as will normally be the case in population or community studies, the weights can be entered into the program, allowing the actual questionnaires to be scored 1 for an affirmative response and 0 for a negative response to each item. This maintains ease of scoring, a further requirement for the measure.

One final word should be said about the use of paired comparisons. In every case, n (n-1) paired comparisons are needed, though certain shortcuts are available (Torgeson, op cit). Thus with 15 items, 105 paired comparisons would be necessary. However, Burroughs (1975) considered the technique to be both statistically elegant and powerful, commenting:

> If this forces us to explore with the rapier of 5 items rather than the bludgeon of 100, it may be no bad thing.

It should be noted that this method of weighting statements has been criticised by Kind (1982). His criticisms are that:

1. The judges may not be consistent in their ratings.
2. One item in the sleep section of the NHP is not on the same psychological continuum and has a different standard deviation from the other four statements.
3. Items have similar scale values.
4. There is an alternative statistical model which produces different scale values.

In classical psychological studies, the reliability of judges' ratings is based on the number of circular triads which they produce. Assuming three statements: A, B and C these triads would be of the form; A>B, B>C, A>C. However, it is possible to argue that this situation may well arise where three statements are rated as of similar severity. The number of such triads could probably be reduced by using expert raters but at the cost of losing 'lay' judgements. Omitting the results from those judges who produce a high number of such triads would undoubtedly improve the statistical 'accuracy' of the weightings - but one must ask whether perceptions are entirely logical. Omitting those data would also have the effect of increasing the distance between scale values - perhaps

Developing an Indicator of Perceived Health

unjustifiably. Kind concludes that the data in
question are in fact satisfactorily reliable.

The sleep statement referred to is that which
asks whether tablets are taken to aid sleep. As has
been shown above, all items (including this one)
were produced from interviews with patients and
hence this is seen as a health problem of relevance.
The scale value for this statement does have a
higher standard deviation than the other four,
indicating a greater range in its perceived severity
- again as judged by lay patients. Thus, the same
arguments apply as in (1). The case for retaining
this item is that taking tablets to aid sleep is
perceived as a health problem and also that it does
affect the responses to the other items. If the
medication is effective then other sleep problems
will not be present and alternatively, the
medication may not be sufficient to 'cure' other
sleep problems.

In relation to the similarity of scale values,
Kind again makes the mistake of confusing classical
psychlogical scaling with that discussed in this
chapter. He argues that two items with a similar
weight should not be included in a measure. This is
because when an instrument is designed to measure
one attitude, a similar score would indicate a
similar reflection of the attitude and hence would
result in tautology. In the case of perceived
health, two statements describing very different
problems may well be judged to be of similar
severity by the patient panel.

Kind argues that there are a number of
different scaling models which can be used to
process this type of preference data and in
particular re-analyses the data using the Bradley-
Terry model (Bradley and Terry, 1952). This model
produces scale values more widely spaced than those
derived from Thurstone's model. The existence of
alternative models clearly indicates the need for
statisticians to determine which model is most
appropriate for deriving scale values in paired
comparison studies such as this. The behavioural
scientists remain dependent on the advice of
statisticians. However, this criticism prompted a
closer look at the weighting procedure described
above. The following data were artificially
constructed to consider the method in a more
critical way.

One hundred subjects were asked to rate the
severity of three statements A, B and C, by the
method of paired comparisons. The F Matrix is shown

in Table 5.4 and is constructed in the same way as that in Table 5.1.

The obtained scale values are:

A = 0.21,   B = -0.04   and   C = -0.17

The weights derived from these scale values are:

A = 38.88,   B = 32.26   and   C = 28.85

It should be noted that these weights have a range of only 10.02 (i.e. the largest minus the smallest weight).

Table 5.4: Matrix F - Hypothetical Data showing the Number of Times each of the Statements A, B and C, was judged more severe than the Other Two by 100 Subjects

		Statement Rated More Severe		
		A	B	C
Statement Rated Less Severe	A	–	40	35
	B	60	–	45
	C	65	55	–

The same hundred subjects were then asked to rate the severity of three further statements : D, E and F. Table 5.5 shows the F Matrix for these judgements. It can be seen that for these three statements the judges were more in agreement about the order of severity with, for example, 90 per cent rating statement D more severe than statement F.

The scale values for these three statements are:

D = 0.65,   E = 0.00   and   F = -0.65

Table 5.5: Matrix F - Hypothetical Data showing the Number of Times each of Three Further Statements, D, E and F, was judged More Severe than the Other Two by the same 100 Subjects.

	Statement Rated More Severe		
	D	E	F
Statement Rated Less Severe D	-	25	10
E	75	-	25
F	90	75	-

and the weights calculated as before are:

D = 49.32,   E = 33.33 and F = 17.34

It should be noted that the range for these weights is 31.98 (49.32 - 17.34).

The weights for statements D to F clearly reflect the greater range of severity as judged by the hundred subjects. This finding suggests that some confidence can be placed in the method of weighting perceived health ' statements described above.

Validity and Reliability

A scale possesses validity when it actually measures what it claims to measure. This immediately leads to problems, as it implies that some independent measure exists with which it can be compared. If this were the case, there would be no point in developing a new test. Thus the ideal form of validation, 'independent criteria', is very difficult to achieve. This is particularly true in the area of subjective health.

Another method is 'logical validation' or 'face validity'. This is the method most commonly used and also the least useful. Basically, face validity means that the measure appears to be achieving what it is designed to. However, if one considers an item such as, 'I cannot run more than 100 yards', one might assume that an affirmative response indicates lack of physical fitness. However, it is possible to suggest conditions where it does not act in that way. For example, it is of little value in assessing the physical fitness of a 90 year old or of someone who has had a leg amputated, or who is confined to a wheelchair. It is of more relevance to a 1,000 meter runner than it is to a weight-lifter, both of whom might consider themselves to be physically fit. An item such as, 'I wake up in the early hours of the morning' is no indication of a perceived health problem for someone who starts work at 5 a.m. Only slightly superior to face validity, is 'jury opinion' in which experts are used to determine the validity of a scale. In the case of the NHP it is difficult to say who could be called an expert in perceived health, and in any case 'juries' were used at each stage of its development.

The most useful technique for validating perceived health measures is probably 'known groups', where validity is implied from the known characteristics of contrasting groups. However, problems still remain. There may be differences between groups which are being compared, other than the variable(s) one is interested in. For example: age, social class, type of housing or available resources, including those of the spouse, may influence responses. A second problem (in the case of the NHP) is that groups are at least partly defined by objective health. Third, people are able to adapt their health problems in such as way as to limit their lifestyle to their capabilities. Someone who suffers pain when walking may decide to give up walking and consequently not perceive him/herself to have that problem.

It might appear obvious that scores should closely reflect clinical assessments. However, if this were the case there would be little point in measuring 'subjective health' and attention should be given to developing a questionnaire which asked about specific symptoms, from which (at least in theory) clinical diagnoses could be made, or perhaps time saved in consultations. However, we have already seen that subjective health status is not the same as objective health status, though they will clearly be related to some extent.

A number of studies which were carried out to validate the NHP, using different approaches, will now be described.

Developing an Indicator of Perceived Health

The first validation study looked at the subjective health of elderly people (Hunt, McKenna, McEwen, Backett and Williams, 1980). The NHP at a minimal level had to be able to distinguish between different degrees of health. Thus groups of subjects were selected who were thought to differ in health status. The elderly were selected for a number of reasons. Earlier work had shown that they have unmet physical, social and emotional needs (Williamson, 1966), and have a tendency to under-report problems to professional agencies, seeing their discomforts as natural concomitants of ageing (Anderson, 1976; Shanas, Townsend, Friis, Nichol and Stenhoumer, 1968; Rudd, 1967). Indeed Linn (1976) had called for the development of an instrument which would allow the identification of elderly people who might need medical or social help or both and those whose problems are due to normal 'healthy' ageing. A further important reason for selecting the elderly in establishing the value of the NHP was that the over-sixties would be the age group most likely to have difficulty in understanding and responding to statements, thereby providing a more severe test of the profile than would groups of younger people.

Four groups of elderly people were selected for study. Group A consisted of 50 men participating in a physical exercise programme and who were judged to be 'fit' and 'active' by physiologists, based on exercise heart rates. Group B included 28 people sampled from a general practitioner's list who had no diagnosed morbidity and who had not consulted their GP in the previous two months. Group C consisted of 49 people who attended a luncheon club run by the social services. The physical health of these subjects varied widely but most had some degree of physical, social or emotional disability. Group D were selected in the same way as Group B but had at least one diagnosed chronic disease which had lasted or would last at least twelve months, the symptoms of which would affect well-being. Eighty six people who satisfied these criteria were approached.

Eighty per cent of subjects contacted agreed to take part and were interviewed at home. Five subjects who had low scores on a short mental status test were omitted. Scores for the four groups showed close similarity between Groups A and B ('low scorers') and Groups C and D ('high scorers') and these groups were combined for the purpose of analysis. Despite the use of the terms 'high-' and 'low-scorers', there was considerable variation in scores within each of the groups. Even with this variance, however, there were clear differences in scores on each of the six sections of the NHP, with the mean scores for Groups A and B all below 5 out of 100, while for Groups C and D the mean scores ranged from about 15 on emotional reactions to about 35 on energy.

Thus the study had gone some way towards establishing convergent construct validity for the Profile, as scores were able to discriminate between people with different health statuses; that is, varying degrees of diagnosed chronic illness and of physical, social and emotional disability, and those who were physiologically fit or who had not recently sought medical intervention.

It would appear from these findings that the congruence between consumer and provider perspectives may be closer than imagined. Patient report is a vital part of individual diagnosis and is likely to play an increasingly important role in the assessment of community needs.

CONSULTERS AND NON-CONSULTERS OF GENERAL PRACTITIONERS

With the exception of preventive measures (immunisation, contraception and ante-natal visits) it can be safely assumed that individuals rarely seek medical advice unless they believe that they have a problem, or for reassurance that they do not. Therefore, whether or not people consult their general practitioner on some medical matter may be seen as an indicator of subjective health status – although the converse is not necessarily true; i.e. that all those who believe themselves to have problems will seek medical attention. Indeed a number of studies have shown that people decide to consult a general practitioner on only a proportion of the occasions on which they suffer complaints. Estimates of the amount of illness that reaches the notice of official health agencies vary from 33 per cent to 50 per cent (Stocks, 1949; Horder and Horder, 1954; Wadsworth, Butterfield and Blaney, 1971; Brotherston, 1958).

Nevertheless, although factors such as the availability of transport, income level and opinions on the efficacy of health services do influence the seeking of health care, the major influence seems to be the individual's perception of his or her health status. For example, studies have shown that patient initiated contacts with the general practitioner do not precisely reflect the presence of morbidity, but rather the differential perception of symptoms (Morrell, 1972). As noted in chapter 4, perceived health status plays an important role in determining whether or not to seek medical care.

Relationships have been found between perceived 'problems' and demands on health services. Greater demands have been found to be made on primary care agencies by patients scoring highly on the Cornell Medical Index than by patients with low scores (Polliack, 1971). Perceived stress amongst students has been shown to be related to the use of college health services (Mechanic and Volkart, 1961) and psychological distress has been shown to be the main variable in both self-rated health and the utilisation of physicians (Tessler and Mechanic, 1978). Studies in London practices have shown that patients who visit the doctor perceive themselves as less healthy and as having more personal problems than do 'self-treaters' (Anderson, Buck, Danaher and Fry, 1977). Finally, it has been found that perception of symptoms and present self-rated health, together with age and sex, are the most important variables influencing the use of medical services (Hannay, 1979).

Perception of health as 'good' does not imply that the individual is symptom free. Dunnel and Cartwright (1972) found the average number of symptoms reported during the previous two weeks was 6.3 for those who considered themselves to be in 'poor' health and 2.4 for those who believed themselves to be in 'excellent' health. Only 4 per cent of the sample reported that they had experienced no symptoms over a four week period.

Reviews of the literature suggest that level of physical activity, time spent away from work or domestic activity due to illness, and overall self-rated health are all indicators of perceived health. The beliefs of the individual about his or her own health act as intervening variables between 'objective' health status and the seeking of medical care. Nevertheless, consulters of the general practitioner may legitimately be supposed to have, in general, a lower subjective health status than non-consulters.

Consequently, a study was carried out to compare scores on the NHP of consulters and non-consulters of general practitioners, controlling for the effects of age and sex. The study also looked at level of physical activity, absence from work or normal daily activity and overall self-rated health status (Hunt, McKenna, McEwen, Williams and Papp, 1981).

A local three-doctor practice with a list size of approximately 9,000 agreed to take part in the study and 100 patient records were extracted at random to estimate mean consultation rate. For the previous year there was a mean combined consultation and repeat prescription rate of 3.88 contacts and it was estimated that 30 per cent of the practice population would have had no contact with a doctor, while 30 per cent would have had three or more contacts in a six month period. For the purpose of the study people who had not consulted a doctor in the previous six months were defined as 'non-consulters', while those who had three or more consultations or repeat prescriptions in the same period were designated 'consulters'. Consultations for contraception, routine medical examinations and innoculations were excluded.

Five hundred and sixty records were extracted representing male and female consulters and non-consulters in the age groups: 20-29, 30-39, 40-49 and 50-59. From these patients, 367 agreed to be interviewed in their homes, a response rate of 70 per cent. Fifteen individuals were not interviewed for administrative reasons. For analysis, an equal number of subjects were assigned to four cells in each age group (male consulters, male non-consulters, female consulters and female non-consulters), with inclusion decided by random sampling. This provided a final sample of 264.

Over 50 per cent of respondents scored zero on each of the sections of the profile and statistical analysis was carried out by non-parametric ranking tests (see section at the end of the chapter on statistical techniques). On every section the consulters scored lower than the non-consulters ($p < 0.01$). No differences in scores were found associated with activity during a normal working day. For activities outside working hours the 'not active' people tended to score higher on energy, pain and physical mobility; but only the difference on energy reached statistical significance. Interestingly, those rated quite active had similar scores to the very active people.

Absence from work or inability to carry out normal daily activities was strongly associated with scores on each section of the profile ($p < 0.001$ in every case). Self-rated health over the past six months and present self-rated health (very good, good, fair or poor) were similarly highly associated with scores on each of the sections ($p < 0.01$ for recent health and $p < 0.001$ for present health).

Females were found to have significantly higher mean scores ($p < 0.05$) on all sections except pain and physical mobility. Differences in scores associated with age were found only on the sleep, social isolation and physical mobility sections.

Given that the decision to consult a doctor for medical reasons is indicative of the perception of a health problem by a patient, this study established criterion validity for the NHP. The sensitivity of the Profile was also confirmed by the fact that the non-consulters did not believe themselves to be problem-free. However, this study, as was the case with all those designed to test reliability and validity, provided interesting findings in itself. The lack of clear cut relationship between amount of physical activity outside work and section scores was not perhaps too surprising in view of the complex relation between activity and feelings of well-being. It is possible that those who undertake a lot of exercise may suffer more problems as a consequence (for example, injuries) than those who take less exercise. This latter group may also worry less about their health and thus perceive themselves as having fewer problems. A number of intervening variables might account for the lack of association between physical activity at work and section scores. People whose jobs involve heavy physical work may be more liable to have accidents, which, whilst not necessarily leading to long absences from work, may give intermittent problems such as back pain or poor sleep. Physical problems may well be less evident in sedentary occupations so that, again, the respondent is less aware of them. Type of work undertaken will be affected by education and socio-economic group, both of which are likely to affect subjective health status. There is a clear need for further study of the association between physical activity and perceived health.

No linear relationship was found between age and scores on the profile. It was the respondents in the 40 to 49 age group who perceived themselves to have most problems. The mid-life transition has been identified as a time when most people become particularly sensitive to their physical, social and emotional states (Stevenson, 1977; Levinson, 1977). As the first signs of ageing become apparent and children grow up, career and domestic roles are called into question and emotional conflict may ensue. Interestingly, it was males in the lower half of the age group who mainly accounted for the higher scores. While some studies have reported higher consultation rates for the elderly, as we have seen above, there is also evidence that as people become older they tend to attribute problems to the ageing process and not to ill health and judge their health against lowered expectations.

The findings that females scored higher on all sections except pain and physical mobility supported earlier studies of sex differences in illness behaviour and the use of health services (Nathanson, 1977) and thus provided a further validation of the Profile. Many reasons can be postulated for the finding. It is possible that females actually experience more distress than males; that they experience the same amount of distress but are more likely to report it; that females are more sensitive to changes in emotional and physiological states. Most studies have found (as in the present study) that women are more likely to report problems in the emotional and social domains, suggesting that there is no general tendency for women to report problems more readily, but that sex differences may lie in differential ability to admit to certain kinds of problems (Mechanic, 1978). The sections of the Profile which showed significant differences between the sexes were those which were the least physical (sleep, energy, emotional reactions and social isolation).

The issues raised by this particular validation study are both numerous and wide-ranging, establishing the value of measures of perceived health in stimulating investigation of the influence of a variety of variables on health care seeking and provision.

STUDIES OF 'FIT' POPULATIONS

Two further validation studies were carried out on 'fit' populations, i.e. groups of people who would be expected to obtain low scores on the Profile. The groups selected for study were firemen and mine rescue workers.

1. Firemen
    With the co-operation of the Nottingham Fire

Department, a list of all active firemen in
Nottinghamshire was obtained. From this list a
random sample of 200 men was selected, each of whom
was sent a postal questionnaire containing the
profile statements. 158 completed profiles were
returned, a response rate of 79 per cent (McKenna,
Hunt, McEwen, Williams and Papp, 1980).

Active firemen are aged between 18 and 55 years
and are expected to be fit in order to undertake
their duties. From the age of 40, they have
medicals every three years. All officers are
encouraged to take part in sports and other forms of
physical exercise and to stay away from work if they
are at all unfit.

On the sections most closely related to
physical fitness; physical mobility and pain, the
mean scores of the firemen were less than 1 out of a
100. For the NHP as a whole the average number of
statements affirmed was only 0.7 per fireman.
However, individual firemen did obtain high scores
on certain sections. For example, on the energy
section one fireman scored 100, while 3 more scored
over 50. Four firemen scored over 50 on the
emotional reactions section and 7 scored over 50 on
the sleep section.

For purposes of comparison the scores of the
firemen were compared with those of the fit elderly
described earlier in this chapter. It is
interesting to note that the mean score of the
firemen was higher on the emotional reactions,
social isolation and sleep sections; while the
firemen scored significantly lower on the pain and
physical mobility sections. Again, it is possible
to postulate that the elderly population have
lowered expectations of their optimum health or that
they have adapted to the health problems which they
do have. A further possibility is that firemen are
more sensitive to their health status, due to the
nature of their work. As we have seen, firemen are
expected to be fit while on duty and are encouraged
to stay away from work when suffering from minor
illnesses which could affect their ability to work
safely.

The high scores obtained by certain firemen
have important implications for industry more
widely. It is well known that the entries in an
accident book give only a partial picture of the
incidence of injury in industry. Similarly, a
great deal of illness never reaches National Health
Service or occupational health service records.
Many workers will experience symptoms which they may

not define as 'illness'. Whether or not an individual seeks medical help is largely a personal decision (as we have seen above) and it is wrong to assume that a worker with an absence of diagnosed illness is fit and healthy. Because of the known association between ill health and increased accident liability and decreased work efficiency, an occupational health nurse who waits in the surgery for an employee to come and seek advice or treatment may be turning a blind eye to the needs of the people in his or her care. Indeed, an unwillingness to admit health problems may well be exacerbated by the present economic situation in which employees may 'hide' ill health rather than risking losing employment when redundancies are feared.

2. Mine rescue workers

Like firemen, mine rescue workers are expected to be fit and healthy. Spencer (1972) stated that the mine rescue worker:

> must be not only in good health but in a state of fitness in which he can withstand severe physical stress.... He should have no physical disability, good muscular power and development and have a full and thorough range of movement of bones and joints.

It was for these reasons that mine rescue workers were selected for study, the expectation being that they would obtain low scores on the NHP (McKenna, Hunt and McEwen, 1981).

The sample consisted of 113 full time miners who were also members of their collieries' mine rescue team. Interviews took place at the collieries and the miners were fit and well enough to work at the time of interview. The respondents completed the NHP on their own and were then asked supplementary questions by specially trained occupational health nurses. In particular, they were asked to rate their present health on a 5 point scale and about any absences from work in the previous six months.

As expected, very few statements in the NHP were affirmed, the mean being 0.56 and the maximum 9 out of 38 statements. Thus, for this group also, the NHP reflected the good health and fitness of the population study group. Once again other interesting findings were made, particularly with respect to health service contact and absence from work.

No differences were found between the number of statements affirmed by miners of different age groups, marital status or number of general practitioner consultations. However, there was a significant difference between the number of statements affirmed and whether or not miners had had repeat prescriptions (p < 0.01).

Table 5.6 shows the types of absence from work reported by the miners. Of the sample 48.7 per cent had had no absence and only one miner had experienced both illness and injury absence.

A chi square test on the data in Table 5.6

Table 5.6: Types of Absence from Work experienced by Mine Rescue Workers in the Previous Six Months		
	No Illness Absence	Had Illness Absence
No Injury Absence	55 (48.7%)	37 (32.7%)
Had Injury Absence	20 (17.7%)	1 (0.9%)

indicated that the two types of absence were not related since those who had sickness absence were unlikely to have injury absence and vice versa (p < 0.02). The mean absences were 3.37 days per six months due to illness and 1.88 days per six months as a result of injury. On a yearly basis this represents a mean total absence of 10.5 days, which is relatively high.

No difference in number of NHP statements affirmed was found between miners who had or had not been absent from work. This finding appeared to obscure the true situation. Miners whose absence was a result of injury affirmed 0.2 statements on average, while the mean number of statements affirmed by miners who had been absent due to illness was 0.92, which was significantly higher than the number affirmed by miners who had no absence (p < 0.05).

Similarly, those miners who had had illness

absence, rated their general health worse than those
who had not been absent in the previous six months
$(p < 0.02)$.

In view of the generally high levels of absence
it was interesting to find only one miner who had
been absent both as a result of illness and
following injury. This supports Hill and Trist's
(1962) withdrawal theory which suggests that the
need for an absence from work is the crucial factor
and that whether this results from ill health or
injury is irrelevant. Certainly, as was discussed
above, except in the case of serious illness or
injury, whether or not to absent oneself from work
is largely the decision of the individual.

Why should the NHP distinguish between people
who have experienced injuries and people who have
been ill? A number of possibilities exist:

1. Healthy people are more likely to have
injuries. This would seem unlikely as the
whole sample was 'fit' and 'healthy' at
the time of the interview.
2. People do not see injuries as a health
problem. Thus the presence (say) of a
broken arm does not lead to a change in
perceived health status. This explanation
is contradicted by evidence presented
later in this chapter.
3. An individual is more willing to absent
himself following injury because it is
'objective', i.e. there for anyone to see
- and probably also entered in the
accident book.
4. Return to work following injury is after
complete recovery, whilst return to work
following illness may be before all
symptoms have completely disappeared. A
few miners with recent illness would
certainly increase the mean number of
statements affirmed by such a 'healthy'
group, if this were the case.
5. People may not consider 'present' health
to be health at the time of answering the
questions but think how their health has
been over the last few weeks or months.
6. Different people tend towards different
type of absence. The theory of accident
proneness has been largely discredited
(see, for example, Hale and Hale, 1971)
although it is recognised that individuals
may go through periods during which they

experience a relatively large number of accidents. Frogatt (1970) has proposed that it is possible to distinguish 'absence prone' individuals who are exhibiting a desire to work discontinuously.

The relationship between illness absence and scores on the NHP does suggest that absence is related to ill health, perhaps to a greater extent than is suggested by the literature (see for example, Taylor, 1968). However, the relation may be with perceived ill health rather than with objective morbidity and perhaps more in the areas of emotional and social functioning.

THE DEVELOPMENT OF PART II OF THE NOTTINGHAM HEALTH PROFILE

At this point in the development of the NHP it was felt that it would be helpful to have additional information on how perceived health problems were affecting daily living. This would add a further dimension referring to functional capacity to augment the data on 'experiential health' (Kelman, 1975). Reference was made to the original statements collected by Martini and McDowell. These were sifted to extract those areas of 'task performance' most often reported to be affected by health problems.

Item analysis established the following activities as being most commonly mentioned:

    Job of work
    Housework
    Social life - e.g. seeing friends, going to
                   the pub
    Family life - relationships with others in the
                   home
    Sex   - intimate relations, love life
    Spare time   - sports, arts and crafts
    activities
    Holidays and travel

Interviews were conducted with patients attending out-patient clinics in the hospital. These interviews confirmed the comprehensiveness of the seven areas, but brought to light a number of difficulties in wording and presentation. For example, not everyone had a family life, or a job.

Housework was considered to be 'sexist'. Sex was thought to be too explicit and narrowly physical, i.e. not including other aspects of the relationship. It was not clear whether job of work included voluntary work.

Further interviews were carried out in hospital clinics, at the Family Planning Clinic and with a variety of university staff from lecturers to canteen assistants. The total number of interviews was 114.

Analysis of these interviews led to revision of the wording of the content areas in an attempt to make them both more comprehensive and more accept-able to respondents. However, it must be admitted that the final version is something of a compromise, as it proved impossible to encompass the complexity of some of the activities in a short and simple questionnaire.

Thus, the content of Part II now refers to:

Job of work, i.e. paid employment

Looking after the home (examples: cleaning and cooking, repairs, odd jobs around the home)

Social life, i.e. going out, seeing friends, going to the pub

Home life, i.e. relationships with other people in the home

Sex life

Interests and hobbies, for example, sports, arts and crafts, do-it-yourself, etc

Holidays, (examples: summer or winter holidays, weekends away)

Clearly, there is still room for ambiguity and there would be people for whom some items would not apply - paid employment, sex life, home life. Adding a third scoring category of 'does not apply' was seriously considered, but eventually rejected as likely to create even more problems of inter-pretation and increase the possibility of errors in response.

Whilst recognising that conceptually Part II was very different from Part I, it was decided to try and obtain weights for the seven activities. Disruption of some areas might have more severe implications than interference with other areas.

Several possible ways of weighting were considered. Finally three different questionnaires were produced.

One required respondents to rank the areas in

order of importance to themselves.
One required respondents to assign a number to each area according to its importance 'in life'.
One utilised the 'anchor' method of assigning an arbitrary value of 100 to one of the areas (home life) and asked people to place all the the other areas on a scale in relation to the anchor point.

Each of these questionnaires was used in conjunction with Part I of the Profile in interviews with 104 people, 60 females and 44 males in the age range 20-70 drawn from clinics, canteens, libraries and relatives of patients.
The results of this exercise showed that people found judging the comparative importance of the areas to be a difficult, if not meaningless, task and there was an enormous variability in allocated ranks for all three questionnaires. However, there was found to be a relatively high correlation ($r = 0.7$) between the number of items affirmed as being affected by health and scores on Part I of the NHP.
It was decided that weighting the seven areas would probably have no advantages over merely summing the numbers of activities affected, to give a crude measure of disruption of task performance. The current version of Part II then, merely requires respondents to answer 'yes' or 'no' to each item and the number of 'yes' responses are added together to give a score between 0 and 7. However, where groups are being compared it is also feasible to take the percentage of the group reporting disruption in each separate activity.

Patients Recoving From Fractures
Complete now with Part II a study was undertaken on the NHP in order to test whether the Profile could detect improvements in health where these might reasonably be expected to occur. Once again it was necessary to select a study population which was likely to obtain relatively high scores on the first occasion. For these reasons, patients who had recently sustained fractures were selected for study (McKenna, McEwen, Hunt and Papp, 1984).
The treatment of many fractures can be seen as involving relatively straightforward clinical procedures. However, the impact of the injury on a patient and the people with whom he or she interacts may present rather more complex problems. In

general, a fracture begins to heal as soon as the bone is broken, and providing the conditions are favourable, healing proceeds through a number of stages until the bone is consolidated (Adams, 1968). For adults, consolidation of a fractured long bone takes about three months, although it can take longer, particularly in the case of bones which have been weakened by disease. Cobey, Cobey, Weil, Greenwald and Southwick (1976) suggested that other factors; social and psychological, might also influence recovery following fractures. They found that the recovery of elderly patients who had suffered a fracture of the hip was influenced by emotional status and degree of social isolation (possibly as much as by the treatment itself). They argued that more specific measures of socio-psychological functioning should be employed in any thorough study of the results of trauma.

In the present study, the experimental group consisted of patients attending a fracture clinic, generally on the day following their injury. The subjects had to meet the following criteria:

1. That they were married or living as married.
2. That they had straightforward fractures, judged by clinic staff as likely to be healed within three months.
3. That they were free from any diagnosed disease thought likely to affect recovery.

A quasi-control group was also employed consisting of the spouses of the experimental subjects. This group was used to control for changes in life-style or home circumstances and also to see whether their perceived health was affected by the injury to their husband or wife. Only those patients whose spouse was willing to take part were included in the study.

Patients who agreed to participate were given NHP's for themselves and their spouses to complete and return in separate reply-paid envelopes. Where both had been returned, each was sent a second Profile to complete eight weeks later.

Over nine weeks, 240 patients and their spouses were given Profiles at the fracture clinic. Of these, 167 (69.6 per cent) completed pairs of Profiles were returned. 141 pairs of subjects returned completed usable Profiles on the second occasion. This represented a secondary response rate of 84.4 per cent or 58.8 per cent of those contacted originally. No statistically significant age or sex differences were found and the data were amalgamated for data analysis. As was discussed earlier in the chapter, age and sex difference on the NHP tend to be masked by the presence of relatively severe morbidity. Table 5.7 shows the mean score of experimental and control subjects on both administrations of Part I of the Profile.

Statistical analysis showed that for the fracture patients there was a significant improvement ($p < 0.001$) in perceived health on all sections except emotional reactions. For the control group the only statistically significant change was in social isolation where problems were greater on the second occasion ($p < 0.05$).

Table 5.7: Fracture Study: Mean Scores of the Experimental and Control Groups on the Six Sections of Part I of the NHP for both Administrations

Section	Experimental group (n=141)		Control group (n=141)	
	1st Admin	2nd Admin	1st Admin	2nd Admin
Pain	26.6	8.0	5.2	6.2
Physical mobility	27.6	6.3	4.8	5.1
Energy	28.8	15.0	17.6	16.7
Sleep	28.0	15.9	12.3	12.4
Social isolation	8.0	3.5	3.5	5.7
Emotional reactions	13.7	10.8	11.0	11.8

Table 5.8 shows the results of the two administrations of Part II of the NHP.

The McNemar test for the significance of changes was used to test whether there were statistically significant differences in the number of subjects changing from affirming to non-affirming the statements and vice versa. Fewer fracture patients claimed to be affected in areas of life ($p < 0.05$ for relationships at home; $p < 0.001$ for all other areas). Again there was one significant

Table 5.8: Fracture study: Number of subjects perceiving areas of life affected by health problems on each administration of Part II of the NHP.

Areas of life	Experimental group (n=141)		Control group (n=141)	
	1st Admin (%)	2nd Admin (%)	1st Admin (%)	2nd Admin (%)
Job of work	74 (52)	26 (18)	9 (6)	12 (9)
Jobs around the home	101 (72)	39 (28)	15 (11)	16 (11)
Social life	56 (40)	14 (10)	9 (6)	16 (11)
Home life	20 (14)	11 (8)	10 (7)	9 (6)
Sex life	46 (33)	22 (16)	21 (15)	28 (20)
Hobbies	92 (65)	43 (30)	14 (10)	20 (14)
Holidays	47 (33)	12 (9)	9 (6)	11 (8)

change for the control group, with an increase in the number of spouses claiming that their social life was adversely affected by their health.

The study clearly showed that the NHP was able to determine improvements in the perceived health of patients recovering from fractures – a group whose 'objective' health status had also improved. However, it provided a much more informative view of the way in which perceived health had changed. The health problems were not confined to the mainly physical aspects of the condition but social integration and other psycho-social aspects of life were also impaired. It is interesting to note that all aspects of life covered by Part II of the NHP were adversely affected and not just those such as work, hobbies and sports.

The one section of Part I where there was no statistically significant improvement in the scores of the fracture sample was emotional reactions, where while 33 per cent had improved scores, 23 per cent had higher scores on the second occasion. Clearly, a relatively high proportion of the patients had worse psychological health associated with recovery from their own injury. This finding may be the result of the long period of disruption to life experienced by many of the experimental

112

group - unable to work or take part in sports and
hobbies. It is also interesting that there was an
increase in the social isolation score of the
control group and in the number who claimed that
their social life was being disrupted at the time of
the second administration of the NHP. These
findings suggest that control subjects suffer
indirectly from their spouses' injuries, possibly as
a result of the disruption caused to their life by
the unscheduled and possibly unwelcome presence of
their spouse. If this is the case, it has important
implications for all carers of handicapped individ-
duals - usually spouses or other family members.

Reliability Testing

A scale or measure is reliable when it will
consistently produce the same results when applied
to the same subjects. Three methods of measuring
reliability are commonly used; multiple form, split-
half and test-retest. In addition, tests of
internal consistency based on statistical models are
becoming more widely used.

1. Multiple form reliability, also known as
   alternate forms, is used where two
   instruments, which have been developed in
   parallel and which measure the same
   attribute, are administered and the scores
   on each instrument correlated. A high
   correlation coefficient would indicate a
   reliable test. However, this method
   obviously necessitates at least twice as
   much work, or two forms of the same
   measure consisting of fewer items.

2. Split-half reliability is a method of
   assessing internal consistency where items
   on an instrument are divided into two
   equivalent parts and correlations between
   the scores on each part are computed.
   This method requires that items in the
   instrument should be homogeneous with
   respect to the attribute being measured,
   and the technique is most useful where a
   large pool of items are used to measure
   only one attribute, for example, in the
   study of attitudes. Two requirements must
   be met; that there is an empirical
   demonstration that the scale is a unity,
   and that each half must contain sufficient
   items to be reliable in itself.

3.   Test-retest reliability. Here the test is
administered to the same population on two
occasions   and   the   results   compared,
usually   by some form of correlation.   Two
problems   are   associated   with this   form
of   reliability   testing.   First,   the
administration of the measure on the first
occasion   may   influence   responses on the
second adminstration.
      Second,   there may be real changes in
the   attribute   being measured between the
two   administrations,   which would lead to
an underestimate of the true reliability.

The   NHP   does   not   meet the requirements for
alternate   form   or   split-half reliability, leaving
only test-retest reliability.

In   order   for an instrument to be trustworthy,
any   changes   in scores over time should be directly
attributable   to   real changes in the variable being
measured, ie changes in perceived health in the case
of   the   NHP.   Other variance will occur as a result
of   experimental error which may take various forms.
For   example,   in   a community study, error variance
would   arise   where a normally healthy individual is
suffering   some acute disease or recent injury.   His
or her scores on the NHP would be higher than normal
and   for   that   individual   would   be   'unreliable'.
However,   in   a   study with a large sample size, one
would   expect   a   certain   proportion of subjects to
have   such temporarily raised scores and it would be
assumed   that   the   proportion   of   such respondents
would   be   the   same   whenever the study was carried
out.

However,   error   variance   may   not   occur
independently and at random.   For   example,   the
initial   completion   of   a   test   may   sensitise the
respondents to the   content   and affect subsequent
administrations.   A   respondent   may try to remember
the   way   he or she answered the questions initially
or   in   a 'before and after' study try to guess what
the researcher wants to hear and answer accordingly.
Similarly,   some   respondents   may   simply   answer
questions at random,in which case the responses will
be neither valid nor reliable.

Earlier   studies   reporting   the reliability of
mailed   questionnaires   concerned with health status
have   been   carried   out, but dealt with illness and
symptoms   rather than health perception (Meltzer and
Hochstim,   1970;   US   National Health Survey, 1960).
The   latter   study   suggested   that negative answers

were more consistent than affirmative ones. Since
the NHP yields a high proportion of negative answers
in 'normal' populations, a test of its reliability
had to be carried out on a population which could be
expected to give a high proportion of affirmative
responses, in order to avoid over-estimating its
reliability. However, for reasons considered above,
the sample would need to be such that the condition
of the respondents would not be expected to change
significantly over a short period of time.

For these reasons patients suffering from
osteoarthrosis were selected for study - specifically those awaiting hip replacement operations
(Hunt, McKenna and Williams, 1981). Osteoarthrosis
is a degenerative bone condition leading to a
chronic state in which there is little change over a
period of weeks, especially when the condition has
become severe enough to warrant arthroplasty.
Osteoarthrosis has implications for the whole
lifestyle of the patient due to the limitations it
imposes on independence and mobility. Surveys of
arthritic patients have described the physical,
social and emotional concomitants of the disease in
terms of pain, disability, restriction of daily
activities and travel, frustration, social isolation
and lack of energy (Chamberlain, Buchanan and Hanks,
1979; McDowell, Martini and Waugh, 1978). It has
been found that the frequency of such complaints is
consistent over the period of a month, although
showing minor variations from day to day (Lunghi,
Miller and McQuillan, 1978). It was for these
reasons that a group of patients with osteoarthrosis
were ideal for testing the reliability of the NHP.

The co-operation of eight orthopaedic surgeons
in the Nottingham area was obtained and access
gained to the lists of patients awaiting arthroplasty of the hip. Patients were selected using the
following criteria - that they had no known
additional conditions or complications which might
affect their health status and that they would not
be likely to be called for their operation during
the period of the study.

A list of the selected patients was sent to the
consultant concerned so that he could verify that
the patients fulfilled these criteria and that they
would not be likely to be distressed by the study.

The number of subjects obtained in this way was
73. Each person was sent the Nottingham Health
Profile, a covering letter, and a pre-paid reply
envelope. All subjects who responded were sent a
second questionnaire four weeks later. The period

of four weeks was chosen in order to reduce over-
estimation of reliability due to memory effects.
Patients were assured of confidentiality and it
was emphasised that their responses would in no way
affect their position on the waiting list.

Fifty eight respondents completed and returned
NHP's on the two occasions (representing an initial
response rate of 88 per cent, of whom 90 per cent
also completed the second questionnaire). As
expected, high scores were obtained on the sections
in Part I. There was also a large number of
affirmative answers to Part II of the NHP,
indicating that health problems were affecting
different aspects of functioning.

Part I of the Profile was tested for reliability using the Spearman correlation coefficient.
Table 5.9 shows the mean score and correlation
coefficient obtained for each of the sections in
Part I.

Perfect reliability would be indicated by a
correlation of 1.0. However, correlations of the
order of 0.8 are relatively rare and very high for
social scientific research of this nature.

As Part II of the NHP provides categorical
data, Cramer's modification of the contingency
coefficient (which allows C to attain unity) was
employed to measure the reliability of responses
(Cramer, 1946; Kendall and Stuart, 1969). Table
5.10 shows the percentage of affirmative responses
to statements on Part II of the NHP and the
associated correlation coefficients.

Table 5.9: Reliability Study: Mean Scores and
Correlation Coefficients on Each Section of Part I
for Patients with Osteoarthrosis (*p < 0.001).

Section of NHP	Mean score (out of 100)	Value of Spearman's
Energy	63.2	0.77*
Pain	70.8	0.79*
Emotional reactions	21.3	0.80*
Sleep	48.7	0.85*
Social isolation	12.5	0.78*
Physical mobility	54.8	0.85*

The correlations between responses on the two administrations of the NHP were thus found to be significantly and satisfactorily high - indicating good reliability. The levels of reliability obtained compare well with other established measures of health status such as the Sickness Impact Profile (Pollard, Bobbitt, Bergner, Martin and Gilson, 1976) and the McMaster Health Index Questionnaire (Chambers and West, 1978) and with widely used intelligence tests such as the Wechsler Adult Intelligence Scale (Wechsler, 1958) and the Stanford-Binet test (Terman and Merrill, 1937).

Table 5.10: Reliability Study: Percentage of Affirmative Responses to Statements on Part II of the NHP and Associated Correlation Coefficients for Patients with Osteoarthrosis ($*p < 0.001$).

Area affected	Affirmative responses (%)	Cramer's C
Paid employment	25.8	0.86*
Jobs around the home	75.8	0.85*
Social life	50.0	0.59*
Family relationships	18.9	0.64*
Sex life	32.7	0.84*
Hobbies/interests	70.6	0.44*
Holidays	67.0	0.71*

This study performed three important functions. First, it established that the NHP was a reliable measure of perceived health. Second, it showed that the measure could be used by post with a high response rate. Finally, it established the potential value of the measure in population studies of patients.

CONCLUSIONS

Chapters 3 and 4 set out the requirements of an indicator of perceived health and this chapter has looked at some of the theoretical issues involved. In order to illustrate practical aspects, the development of the Nottingham Health Profile has been described and it is now possible to see how far this measure satisfies the stated criteria.

The main aim was to develop a measure of perceived health and this was done by gathering statements about the impact of ill health from lay people - avoiding clinical judgements. Lay judges were also used in the process of weighting statements to reflect the perceived severity of each item in a section.

A further advantage of using non-professionals in the development of the NHP was that the symptoms were not included in the measure. This has the effect of allowing people to complete the Profile who have not been labelled unhealthy or who do not consider themselves ill. Thus individuals who rate their health good may still find statements which are appropriate to them. Avoiding the use of medical terms also frees the respondent from thinking and replying in the language of physicians.

The NHP is short, easily administered and completed and is readily understood, requiring only a low reading age. It has been shown to be completely satisfactory for a wide variety of groups of subjects, including the frail and elderly. While only requiring a yes/no response to each of the 38 statements, these items have been weighted to reflect the perceived severity of each, adding greater meaning to the measure as a whole.

The NHP measures areas of experience which are susceptible to change and consequently is able to monitor the effects of interventions as well as the health of populations. In addition, the measure provides a comprehensive picture of individual patterns of perceived ill-health providing information on both physical and psycho-social health problems.

Scores on the Profile are expressed in an easily interpretable way. All sections of Part I are scored out of 100 and these scores can be presented in the form of bar charts, allowing visual comparison of perceived health problems in each of the six sections. Responses to the Profile are easily scored, especially with the aid of a computer (essential where population studies are being undertaken). No sophisticated mathematical or computing skills are required and the data are readily handled by the standard statistical packages. Finally, scores on the NHP can readily be analysed in relation to other variables of interest such as sex, age, social class.

Thus it can be seen that the final version of the NHP and the associated weights for each statement meet the requirements of a perceived health measure discussed in the previous two chapters. The following chapter shows how norms have been generated for this version of the NHP an essential stage in the development of a research instrument.

REFERENCES

Adams, J.C. (1968) Fractures, 5th edition, Livingstone, Edinburgh

Anderson, J.A.D. Buck, C. Danaher, K. and Fry, J. (1977) 'Users and Non-Users of Doctors: Implications for Self Care', Roy Coll Gen Pract, 27, 155-159

Anderson, W.F. (1976) 'Preventive Aspects of Geriatric Medicine', Physiotherapy, 62, 146-148

Barrett, M. (1914) 'A Comparison of the Order of Merit Method and the Method of Paired Comparisons', Psychol Rev, 21, 278-294

Beck, A.T. Ward, C.H. Mendleson, M.J. and Erbaugh, J. (1961) 'An Inventory for Measuring Depression', Archs Gen Psychiat, 4, 53-63

Bradley, R.A. and Terry, M.E. (1952) 'Rank Analysis of Incomplete Block Designs. 1. The Method of Paired Comparisons', Biometrika, 39, 324-345

Brotherston, J.H.F. (1958) 'Some Factors affecting the Use of G.P. Services on a Housing Estate near London', in J. Pemberton and H. Willard (eds.), Recent Studies in Epidemiology, Oxford University Press, London

Burroughs, G.E.R. (1975) Design and Analysis in Educational Research, (2nd Edition), Educational Monograph, No. 8, Educational Review, Oxford

Chamberlain, M.A. Buchanan, J.M. and Hanks, H. (1979) 'The Arthritic in an Urban Environment', Anns Rheum Dis, 38, 51-56

Chambers, L.W. and West, A.E. (1978) 'The St John's Randomised Trial of the Family Practice Nurse: Health Outcomes of Patients', Int J Epidemiol, 7, 153-161

Cobey, J.C. Cobey, J.H. Conant, L. Weil, U.H. Greenwald, W.F. and Southwick W.O. (1976) 'Indicators of Recovery from Fractures of the Hip', Clinical Orthopaedics, 117, 258-262

Conklin, E.S. (1923) 'The Scale of Values Method for

Studies in Generic Psychology', University of Oregon Publications, 2, No. 1

Conklin, E.S. and Sutherland, J.W. (1923) 'A Comparison of the Scale of Values Method with the Order of Merit Method', J Exp Psychol, 6, 44-57

Cramer, H. (1946) Mathematical of Statistics, Princeton University Press, Princeton

Dunnell, K. and Cartwright, A. (1972) Medicine Takers, Prescribers and Hoarders, Routledge and Kegan Paul, London

Frogatt, P. (1970) 'Short Term Absence from Industry. III. The Inference of "Proneness" and a Search for Causes', Brit J Indust Med, 27, 297-312

Goldberg, D. (1972) The Detection of Psychiatric Illness by Questionnaire, Oxford University Press, London

Goode, W.J. and Hatt, P.K. (1952) Methods in Social Research, McGraw-Hill, New York, p. 286

Hale, A.R and Hale, M. (1971) 'Accidents in Perspective', Occup Psychol, 44, 115-118

Hannay, D. (1979) 'Factors associated with Formal Symptom Referral', Soc Sci Med, 13A, 101-107

Hill, J.J.M. and Trist, E.L. (1962) Industrial Accidents, Sickness and Other Absences, Tavistock, London

Horder, J. and Horder, E. (1954) 'Illness in General Practice', Practitioner, 173, 177-179

Horst, A.P. (1941) 'The Prediction of Personal Adjustment', Social Science Research Council Bulletin, No. 48

Hunt, S.M. McKenna, S.P. McEwen, J. Backett, E.M. Williams, J. and Papp, E. (1980) 'A Quantitative Approach to Perceived Health Status: A Validation Study', J Epidemiol Comm Hlth, 34, 281-286

Hunt, S.M. McKenna, S.P. McEwen, J. Williams, J. and Papp, E. (1981) 'The Nottingham Health Profile: Subjective Health Status and Medical Consultations', Soc Sci Med, 15A, 221-229

Hunt, S.M. McKenna, S.P. and Williams, J. (1981) 'Reliability of a Population Survey Tool for Measuring Perceived Health Problems. A Study of Patients with Osteoarthrosis', J Epidemiol Comm Hlth, 35, 297-300

Kelman, S. (1975) 'The Social Nature of the Definition Problem in Health', Int J Hlth Servs, 5, 625-642

Kendall, M.G. and Stuart, A. (1969) The Advanced Theory of Statistics, Vol. 2. Inference and

Relationship, 3rd ed Griffin, London

Kind, P. (1982) 'A Comparison of Two Models for Scaling Health Indicators', Int J Epidemiol, 11, 271-275

Levinson, D.J. (1977) 'The Mid-Life Transition: A Period in Adult Psychosocial Development', Psychiat, 40, 99-106

Likert, R. (1932) 'A Technique for the Measurement of Attitudes', Arch Psychol, No. 140

Linn, M.W. (1976) 'Studies in Rating the Physical, Mental and Social Dysfunction of the Chronically Ill Aged', Medical Care, 14, suppl 119-126

Lunghi, M.E. Miller, P.M.C. and McQuillan, W.M. (1978) 'Psycho-social Factors in Osteo-arthritis of the Hip', J Psychosom Res, 22, 57-63

McDowell, I. and Martini, C.J.M. (1976) 'Problems and New Directions in the Evaluation of Primary Care' Int J Epidemiol, 5, 247-250

McDowell, I. Martini, C.J.M. and Waugh, W. (1978) 'A Method of Self Assessment of Disability before and after Hip Replacement Operations', Brit Med J, 2, 875-879

McKenna, S.P. Hunt, S.M. and McEwen, J. (1981) 'Weighting the Seriousness of Perceived Health Problems using Thurstone's Method of Paired Comparisons', Int J Epidemiol, 10, 93-97

McKenna, S.P. Hunt, S.M. and McEwen, J. (1981) 'Absence from Work and Perceived Health among Mine Rescue Workers', J Soc Occup Med, 31, 151-157

McKenna, S.P. Hunt, S.M. McEwen, J. Williams, J. and Papp, E. (1980) 'Looking at Health from the Consumer's Point of View', Occup Hlth, 32, 330-335

McKenna, S.P. McEwen, J. Hunt, S.M. and Papp, E. (1984) 'Changes in the Perceived Health of Patients recovering from Fractures', Pub Hlth, 98, 97-102

Martini, C.J.M. and McDowell, I. (1976) 'Health Status: Patient and Physician Judgements', Health Services Research, 11, 58-515

Martini, C.J.M. and McDowell, I. (1977) 'The Evaluation of Strategies for the Improvement of Life Style: An Example Drawn from two Locomotor Disorders', Paper read at a conference of the International Epidemiological Association, Puerto Rico

Mechanic, D. (1978) 'Sex, Illness Behaviour and the Use of Health Services', Soc Sci Med, 12B, 207-

214

Mechanic, D. and Volkart, E.H. (1961) 'Stress, Illness Behaviour and the Sick Role', Amer Sociol Rev, 26, 51-59

Meltzer, J.W. and Hochstim, J.R. (1970) 'Reliability and Validity of Survey Data on Physical Health', Pub Hlth Reps, 85, 1075-1086

Morrell, D.C. (1972) 'Symptom Interpretation in General Practice', J Roy Coll Gen Pract, 22, 297-300

Mosteller, F. (1951) 'Remarks on the Method of Paired Comparisons. 1. The Least Squares Solution assuming Standard Deviations and Equal Correlations', Psychometrika, 16, 3-11

Nathanson, C.A. (1977) 'Sex, Illness and Medical Care: A Review of Data, Theory and Method', Soc Sci Med 11, 13-25

Osgood, C.E. Suci, G.J. and Tannenbaum, P.H. (1957) The Measurement of Meaning, University of Illinois Press, Urbana

Pollard, W.E. Bobbitt, R.A. Bergner, M. Martin, D.P. and Gilson B.S. (1976) 'The Sickness Impact Profile: Validation of a Health Status Measure', Medical Care, 14, 57-67

Polliack, M.R. (1971) 'The Relationship between Cornell Medical Index Scores and Attendance Rates', J Roy Coll Gen Pract, 21, 453-455

Rudd, T. (1967) Human Relations in Old Age, Faber, London

Scott, C. (1961) 'Research on Mail Surveys', J Roy Stat Soc, 124, 143-205

Shanas, E. Townsend, P. Friis, S. Nichol, P. and Stenhoumer, J. (1968) Old People in Three Industrial Societies, Routledge and Kegan Paul, London

Spencer, T.D. (1972) 'Medical Aspects of Mines Rescue' in J.M. Rogan (ed.), Medicine in the Mining Industries, Heinemann, London

Stevenson, J. (1977) Issues and Crises during Middlescence, Appleton-Century-Crofts, New York

Stocks, P. (1949) Sickness in the Population of England and Wales in 1944-7, General Registry Office of Studies on Medical and Population Subjects, No. 2, HMSO, London

Taylor, P.J. (1968) 'Sickness Absence Resistance', Trans Soc Occup Med, 18, 96-100

Terman, L.M. and Merrill, M.A. (1937) Measuring Intelligence, Houghton, Mifflin, Boston

Tessler, R. and Mechanic, D. (1978) 'Psychological Distress and Perceived Health Status', J Hlth Soc Behav, 19, 254-259

Thurstone, L.L. (1927) 'Psychophysical analysis', Amer J Psychol, 38, 368-389

Thurstone, L.L. (1927) 'A Law of Comparative Judgement', Psych Rev, 34, 273-286

Thurstone, L.L. (1959) The Measurement of Values, University of Chicago Press, Chicago

Torgerson, W.S. (1958) Theory and Methods of Scaling, John Wiley, New York

US National Health Survey (1960) A Study of Special Purpose Medical History Techniques, PHS, Publication No. 584 series D, No. 1 US Government Printing Office, Washington DC

Wadsworth, M.E.J. Butterfield, W.J.H. and Blaney, R. (1971) Health and Sickness: The Choice of Treatment, Tavistock, London

Wechsler, D. (1958) The Measurement and Appraisal of Adult Intelligence, 4th edition Williams and Wilkins, Baltimore

Williamson, J. (1966) Ageing in Modern Society, Paper presented to the Royal Society of Health, Edinburgh, 9th November

Chapter 6.

MEASURING PERCEIVED HEALTH IN THE COMMUNITY

All the studies using the Nottingham Health Profile described so far have involved specially selected groups. However, it will be recalled that the objective was to develop a 'population survey tool'. Hence it was necessary to use the NHP to survey samples of individuals from the population at large.

ESTABLISHING NORMS FOR THE NOTTINGHAM HEALTH PROFILE

The next stage in the development of a measure is to establish norms or marker scores. We already know that mean scores below five on any section of Part I are indicative of a 'healthy' population and that mean scores of around 50 (as found for patients with osteoarthrosis) indicate severe perceived health problems. However, the numbers or scores themselves have no implicit meaning. Meaning can only be inferred where comparisons are made. Hence, firemen are 'healthy' (or more accurately, have a higher perceived health status) as compared to patients with osteoarthrosis and consulters of general practitioners tend to have greater perceived health problems than people who do not seek medical care.
    However, there will be many occasions on which only one group will be studied or assessed. In such a situation the investigator will still need to know what scores would be expected from a group comparable with that being studied. If, for example, one wished to assess perceived health in an inner city population it would be necessary to have some idea of what scores on the NHP an 'average' or 'normal' population would show. Such an 'average' or 'normal' score is a norm - a standard with which scores from subsequent studies can be compared.

124

The development of norms has always been an important part of the development of psychological measures, although it has been largely neglected by the developers of perceived health measures. The best examples of norm development have been intelligence tests. The ubiquitous IQ is primarily an index of rate of intellectual growth and thus a prediction of the ultimate level of 'intelligence' an individual will achieve on maturity (Vernon, 1960). It was originally calculated by relating mental age (MA) to chronological age (CA) thus:

$$IQ = \frac{MA}{CA} \times 100$$

where IQ represents present intelligence level. Of course the equation breaks down as the child reaches adolescence: a child 'two years' ahead of his or her time would have an IQ of 140 at age 5 and only 113 at age 15. To overcome this problem percentiles have been used. For example, it is known that the top 2.5 per cent of children have IQs of 130 plus and that the top 9 per cent obtain 120 plus. By plotting the 97.5 percentile line for each age, a curve can be drawn indicating the score that needs to be achieved by a child of any age to obtain an IQ of 130. In this way the score on the test is determined by a comparison of the individual with his or her peers. Considering perceived health, it would be wrong to compare the score of a group of 60 year olds with a group of 20 year olds, and then attribute the difference to variables such as type of housing or physical activity undertaken. Any difference due to these variables must be determined by comparing the scores of the 60 year olds with those of a random sample of people of a similar age.

Two large scale studies have been carried out to develop norms for the NHP. Both were designed to look at the association between sex, age, social class and scores obtained. The first study was of the general population and the second of employees in a large manufacturing organisation.

Norms for a General Population

The co-operation of a four- doctor group practice near Nottingham was obtained and a random sample of males and females divided into five year age groups from 20 to over 75 years was drawn. Three thousand two hundred questionnaires were sent out and 2,192

(68 per cent) usable profiles were returned after ten weeks. Additional information collected allowed social class to be coded using the British Registrar General's classification, said to be related to 'general standing within the community of the occupations concerned' (Office of Population Censuses and Surveys, 1970). The distribution of the respondents with respect to social class, age, sex, marital status and type of accommodation was compared with data from the 1971 Census (Her Majesty's Stationery Office, 1974). No statistically significant differences were found in social class, sex distribution or marital status. Ages 20-29, 40-45 and over 69 were over-represented in this sample and there were more owner-occupiers and fewer tenants compared with national figures.

These differences and the nature of the town in which the study was undertaken may have led to certain biases in the study. Such biases (should they have occurred) could only be avoided by carrying out a large scale study with respondents sampled at random from the whole of Great Britain or the United Kingdom. However, while such a study would be valuable for looking at national trends, it could be argued that a series of smaller population studies would be more valuable. Such studies might survey inner and outer urban areas, towns and rural areas. Regional studies might also detect differing distributions of perceived health problems.

Readers are referred to Hunt, McEwen and McKenna (1985) for details of scores obtained, but the main findings can be summarised as follows:

1. The relation between perceived health and social class occurs only in the age group 20-24. This has important implications at both a theoretical and practical level for explanations of persisting inequalities in health.

2. Scores on the Profile convey a clear picture of differences in perceived health problems between social classes for these younger age groups.

3. On average, a male in the age range 20-44 and coming from social classes IV and V will score twice as highly as his contemporary from social classes I or II on the energy and emotional reactions section, over 3 times as high on the sleep section and over 4 times as high on feelings of social isolation. These

           scores are shown in Table 6.1.
4.   Similar, though less marked findings occurred for females. Some masking of social class effects may have occurred because of the general tendency of females to score more highly than men.
5.   The lower social classes feel themselves to have a much larger burden of socio-emotional problems than do the others, but this difference becomes less marked after the age of 45.

There are of course several possible explanations of these findings. However, we would argue that the differences noted in the younger age groups reflected a real difference in health between the social classes, with the disappearance of these differences as age increases being primarily accounted for by lowered expectations.

Table 6.1: Norms for a General Population in the East Midlands: Mean scores for Males aged 20-44 Years on Sections of Part I of the NHP, by Social Class.

	Social Class			
	I & II (n=105)	III NM (n=49)	III M (n=102)	IV & V (n=43)
Energy	5.49	4.31	3.58	12.74
Pain	2.05	2.39	3.07	1.03
Emotional reactions	7.54	7.25	8.32	18.25
Sleep	5.63	7.77	7.38	19.17
Social isolation	2.82	2.08	2.77	12.56
Physical mobility	1.46	1.18	0.73	1.76

Younger people may well think in terms of 'bettering' themselves and sufficient class mobility does occur to make this a realistic ambition, although the move is generally only one class upward (Goldthorpe and Llewellyn, 1977). It is conceivable that by the age of 45 most people have adjusted to their position in life and have realistically lowered or achieved their expectations. It seems likely that the early forties represent a crisis point after which resignation and adaptation occur. Financial problems also ease with age when incomes tend to be higher and mortgage or rent payments less of a burden. Children will generally have left home or become self-supporting. In comparison with their earlier life, people will be experiencing a relatively higher standard of living.

A further explanation may be the excess of mortality in classes IV and V in the younger age groups - suggesting that those who survive are likely to be fitter. However, there is a greater prevalence of chronic disease in classes IV and V in older people and this has not shown up in scores on the Profile, probably as a result of lowered expectations and attribution of problems to advancing age.

Results from Part II of the Profile support the general theme of those from Part I, though they are not so clear cut. Men from the lower social classes are significantly more likely to feel the effects of health problems on their daily life, especially paid employment, jobs around the home, social life and holidays. Social class differences do not show up for females, again perhaps because of their tendency to score highly regardless of class. Social class effects in women may also be obscured by the convention of classifying them by their husband's occupation.

Such a discussion of the implications of the study findings illustrates how this routinely collected information can stimulate interest and further research. The main value of the study remains the development of norms with which subsequently collected scores can be compared. Mean scores by age and sex from this study can be found in the Appendix.

It should be noted that the larger the sample sizes employed, the more accurate will be the mean scores (or norms) obtained. For this reason, all researchers using the NHP in community or population studies are encouraged to pass on copies of their data to one of the authors of this book. In this

way more accurate, up to date and wider-ranging
norms can be developed.
    Scores on a measure such as the NHP might well
be expected to be influenced by factors such as
culture, environment and economic climate as well as
the variables known to have a major influence on
health status such as sex, age and social class. A
study discussed later in the chapter provides NHP
data for inner- and outer- boroughs of London.
These urban areas might well be expected to produce
different mean scores on the NHP - even when sex,
age and social class are taken into account.

Adapting Norms for Comparison
Studies using the NHP will have samples differing in
composition, and in order to make comparisons with
the norms it will be necessary to weight them
appropriately. This is a straightforward procedure
and can be illustrated by a hypothetical sample and
the information contained in Table 6.2.
    The hypothetical sample consists of men aged 20
to 44. Twenty of these men are from social classes
I and II, 40 from class III NM, 50 from class II M
and 30 from classes IV and V. For the energy
section, the 'expected' mean score would be:

$$\frac{(20 \times 5.49 + (40 \times 4.31) + (50 \times 3.58) + (30 \times 12.74)}{140}$$

This would give a value of 6.02. The investigator
can now compare any overall mean score for energy

Table 6.2: Hypothetical Data showing Mean Score
on the Energy Section of NHP by Social Class

	Social Class			
	I & II	III NM	III M	IV & V
Energy Section (mean score)	5.49	4.31	3.58	12.74
n	20	40	50	60

with this norm weighted by the social class of the sample. Similarly, a sample can be weighted for age and for sex composition.

Norms for an Employed Population
The study discussed above covered a random population, i.e. all people over the age of 19 registered with a general practitioner. Such a sample will include unemployed and prematurely retired people (under the age of 60 for women or 65 for men) as well as people who are absent from work. Furthermore, a large proportion of the women in the sample will not be employed full time - their social class grouping being dependent on their husband's occupation.

For these reasons separate norms need to be developed for industrial and commercial settings, where many studies of perceived health are likely to be undertaken. In order to develop such norms a study was undertaken in a large company employing a variety of industrial and commercial processes and providing diverse types of employment. Sites within the organisation were selected in order to cover a range of social class groupings.

Ideally, the questionnaires should have been sent to the homes of the sample selected for study. However, the management of the organisation involved did not wish to provide the names and addresses of their employees and suggested that the questionnaires should be distributed internally via the managers in each site. Consequently, the researchers had no control over whether the profiles were actually distributed or not and were unable to issue reminders to non-responders. A total of 3,000 profiles were sent to the firm and 1,753 usable questionnaires were returned; a response rate of 58 per cent, lower than in any other study in which the NHP has been used. It seems likely that a number of people in the sample did not receive a questionnaire and that the response rate quoted is really an underestimate. Because of the anonymity maintained it was not possible to compare responders with non-responders.

Detailed scores can be found in McEwen, Lowe, Hunt and McKenna (1985) but scores for the whole sample by social class are shown in Table 6.3. The data in the table again show the characteristic social class gradients, with employees in social classes IV and V having higher scores. Similar trends were found for Part II and the percentage of

Table 6.3: Norms for an Employed Population in
the East Midlands: Mean Scores on Part I of the
NHP for the Whole Sample, by Social Class

	Social Class				
	I	II	III N	III M	IV & V
Energy	10.2	7.8	12.1	13.8	16.7
Pain	1.4	1.7	2.9	4.3	4.6
Emotional reactions	5.5	5.7	9.5	12.6	14.9
Sleep	6.3	6.4	9.7	14.1	13.8
Social isolation	4.2	5.1	4.2	5.4	8.6
Physical mobility	1.6	1.4	2.3	4.2	3.4

respondents in each social grouping who indicated
that aspects of their life had been adversely
affected by their health are shown in Table 6.4.

Evidence from the study suggested that age,
sex, social class and perceived disability all
influenced scores on the NHP. Detailed analyses
indicated that the effect of these variables when
combined provided a good explanation of the
variations in levels of perceived health.

As expected, mean scores for this employed
sample tended to be lower than those for the general
population. This trend was reversed in a few areas.
For example, male employees tended to score higher
on social isolation problems than did males in the
general practitioner sample. However, within 'the
healthy workforce' there was still an appreciable
number of health problems which affected the full
range of areas of living.

One interesting aspect of this study is the
potential of an occupational health service for
influencing the health of employees; particularly in
health promotion. While the NHP cannot determine
the exact nature of health problems nor their cause,

Table 6.4: Norms for an Employed Population in the East Midlands: Percentages of Employees reporting Areas of their Life affected by Health on Part II of the NHP, by Social Class.

	Social Class				
	I	II	III N	III M	IV & V
Employment	3.4	5.2	7.0	12.4	13.7
Looking after the home	8.1	5.8	7.9	12.0	11.2
Social life	6.0	4.4	7.3	11.6	12.5
Home life	4.7	3.7	6.9	10.4	11.3
Sex life	5.4	4.2	6.0	11.2	9.4
Interests and hobbies	9.4	6.6	7.2	12.0	11.9
Holidays	3.4	4.2	4.5	11.2	10.6

it can indicate that problems exist and encourage participation in health promotion activities. The impact of educational and other measures designed to change behaviour relevant to health could be evaluated by a second administration of the NHP as well as by more objective measures such as tobacco and alcohol consumption and sickness absence. Attempts to establish smoking policies and smoking cessation activities have shown the value of a preliminary questionnaire to all the staff (Perkins, 1984). The Profile might provide such a motivating tool, particularly if used on an individual basis to show how health status has changed as a result of changed behaviour.

Extending and Updating Norms
The two studies just described were designed to develop norms or benchmarks with which subsequent scores on the NHP could be compared. One drawback of the studies is that both were based in the East

Midlands. As was suggested above, there is good reason to suppose that levels of perceived health may vary by region as well as by the variables which were measured; social class, age and sex. The norms can be weighted to make them match the social class, age and sex make-up of the population under investigation but other uncontrolled variables are likely to influence perceived health scores.

Ideally, studies should be carried out in the different regions of England and in Scotland and Wales to determine expected scores in these areas. Similarly, as was stated above, it would seem likely that scores will vary between inner- and outer-city areas, suburbs and rural areas.

Different industrial processes may well be associated with different health problems; for example, exposure to toxic substances or the varying likelihood of occupational trauma. Clerical staff might well have different patterns of health problems from production staff - not necessarily totally accounted for by social class differences.

For these reasons, any measure of perceived health should provide norms for a wide range of populations. Such norms can only be developed if researchers using the measure forward their results for collation by some central agency. Strict anonymity would of course always be maintained by such an agency. In return, the collectors would, upon request, supply other NHP users with the most appropriate set of norms with which to compare their data.

A second important reason for continuing to collect data from populations is that norms may well become outdated. Just as mean height and IQ increase over time, so changes may be expected to occur in perceived health. In the case of IQs they can be continually changed to ensure that the mean is standardised at 100. This is done by basing IQ scores on the 50th percentile or median score. Thus, any individual completing an intelligence test will be compared with the norm for his or her age group based on recent scores - not those obtained 10 or 20 years earlier.

Morbidity within a population is constantly changing and this is likely to lead to changes in perceived health status. While the health of populations in developed countries will improve over time, there are clear cyclical changes over certain time periods. Such variations have been shown to be related to economic changes within society (see for example; Brenner and Mooney, 1983). As we will see below, the health of people who become unemployed tends to deteriorate both for psycho-social and financial reasons. The health of members of the families of unemployed bread-winners also suffers. Given the conservative estimate of over three million people unemployed in Great Britain in 1985, it would not be surprising to find that the overall health of the nation deteriorated over the following few years. In contrast, developments in medical science, while not being able to prevent or cure increasingly prevalent chronic diseases, have managed to reduce the impact of impairments, disabilities and handicaps and hence have improved perceived health status. Consider the impact on perceived health of a cure for osteoarthritis. As we have seen in the previous chapter, patients awaiting replacement hips scored very highly on all sections of the NHP. It follows that new norms will be required in response to changes in the health status of the new population under study.

POPULATION STUDIES EMPLOYING THE NOTTINGHAM HEALTH PROFILE AS AN ESTABLISHED RESEARCH TOOL

This section describes two areas of research in which the NHP has been used both cross-sectionally and longitudinally as an established measure of perceived health. In the first, two populations are compared - inner-city and outer-city boroughs. Findings are then presented from studies in which the NHP was used to compare the perceived health of employed, unemployed and laid-off workers and to measure changes in health status over time within these groups.

Intra-urban Variations in Health
Curtis (1985) undertook a household survey in two boroughs in the North East Thames health region in order to gather data on the health status and use of medical services reported by residents. The boroughs, Tower Hamlets and Redbridge, were typical of inner- and outer-city areas of East London. In particular, the research was designed to study:

1. Self-reported morbidity.
2. Patterns of service use.
3. The local prevalence of morbidity in the community.
4. The association between morbidity and

social deprivation.
5.   The   performance   of   local   medical
     services - especially of primary care.

Self-reported   morbidity   data   were   considered
preferable   to   clinical   assessments   by   medical
personnel   as   they   allowed   the assessment of ill-
health   and   undiagnosed   or   untreated morbidity as
well   as   that   reaching   the   attention   of medical
services.   Self-reported measures have the advantage
of   being   determined   by the patient rather than by
clinical 'objective' diagnoses and of being related
more to impact on function.

Curtis argues that these data:

1.   Are   more   likely   to correspond closely
     to   health   attitudes   and   behaviour   -
     reflecting the individual's propensity and
     motivation   to   improve   their   health   or
     maintain good health.
2.   Are   capable of providing a useful method
     of   assessing   levels   of   need associated
     with   differing   medical   conditions   -
     allowing   the   identification   of priority
     need   groups among those with a variety of
     illnesses.
3.   Are   particularly   valuable   in   measuring
     chronic   illness,   where   health   services
     have   a   role   in   alleviating   suffering
     rather than providing a cure.
4.   Are   readily comprehensible to non-medical
     people - providing greater accountability
     of   resource   allocation   to   the   general
     public - as policy should be a reflection
     of   the   views of society on how resources
     should be apportioned.

However,   it   is   noted   that   while   self-reported
morbidity   can   indicate   likely pressure on general
medical   services   and   the   extent to which service
distribution   between   different   population   groups
corresponds   to   relative   need,   it cannot indicate
what   mode   of   provision   is   likely   to   be   most
effective   in   meeting   these   needs   -   unless   the
measures   are used as part of an evaluative study of
particular   services.   It   is   also pointed out that
the   distribution   of resources will remain a matter
of   policy and of politics.   The overall size of the
resource   'cake'   to be divided will govern the scale
of   service   provision which is possible and this will
determine   what   level   of severity of morbidity (or

135

perhaps which types of morbidity) the health service will aim to alleviate.

Three measures of morbidity were used in the study; questions derived from the General Household Survey; the Nottingham Health Profile and a list of common symptoms. These measures were chosen for the reasons stated above and because they provided data in a standard form for all respondents and permitted comparison with results from other morbidity surveys (i.e. norms for comparison were available). The instruments had the additional advantages of being suitable for a range of different types of respondents and of being acceptable and simple to administer within the interview.

Three hundred households were sampled in each borough. After allowing for ineligible addresses, 'no contacts' and refusals, the response rate was 67 per cent of households in Tower Hamlets and 76 per cent in Redbridge. These figures compare with a 77 per cent response rate in Greater London for the 1981 General Household Survey (Office of Population Censuses and Surveys, 1983).

An analysis was performed to assess the impact of interviewer effects - the extent to which the interviewers themselves influence the responses of the interviewees. This analysis showed that the General Household Survey (GHS) instruments were particularly susceptible to interviewer effects and consequently less reliable as comparative morbidity indicators than the NHP. This finding was important, as observed differences between the boroughs in prevalence of morbidity measured by the GHS may have been spurious, while the NHP results do support the hypothesis that the two boroughs were experiencing differing levels of self-perceived morbidity.

Mean scores on the NHP for the two boroughs are shown in Table 6.5, together with data from inner- and outer-city areas in Manchester (Leavey, 1982).

Analysis of the data from London showed that more morbidity was reported by Tower Hamlets respondents than by those from Redbridge - with the differences being statistically significant, except in the case of sleep problems. These contrasts were strongest in the population below the age of 65. Similar findings were obtained in the Manchester study. In fact, the mean scores obtained in the two studies were remarkably similar - suggesting that greater confidence can be placed in each study and that the obtained scores might be adequate norms for comparisons of inter- and outer-city areas throughout England.

It is interesting to note that the intra-urban contrasts in both cities were less apparent in evidence obtained from OPCS instruments than in the NHP results. Curtis suggested that this may have been due to the NHP's greater sensitivity to variations in morbidity than that of the General Household Survey instruments.

Having established a higher level of morbidity reported by residents in the inner-city area - Curtis then considered the social factors which might account for such differences. In particular, she considered the variables; marital status, occupational class, housing tenure, country of origin and car ownership. All of these factors, except country of origin, were found to be highly associated with NHP scores. Combining data from the two boroughs gave the following findings (with statistical significance assessed by Chi-square at the 5 per cent level):

1. There were significant differences on all sections of the NHP associated with marital status. In all cases except social isolation, single people scored lowest followed by married respondents and finally those respondents who were widowed, divorced or separated. However, it is possible that these differences were inflated by the effects of the sex and age of respondents in each group.

2. For social class, significant differences were found again for all sections of the NHP, with social classes IV and V and the retired having the highest scores.

3. Housing tenure showed significant differences on all sections except emotional reactions and sleep. People in property rented from the council tended to score highest followed by people in privately rented accommodation. Owner occupancy was associated with the lowest scores on the NHP.

4. Again on all sections, those who had a car scored considerably lower than those who did not. It should be noted that both housing tenure and car ownership are good indicators of social class.

Table 6.6 shows the same information for the three age groups studied separately. Asterisks indicate

Table 6.5: Mean NHP Scores for Respondents in Inner- and Outer-city Areas of London and Manchester

NHP Section	Age	Inner London	Outer London	Inner Manchester	Outer Manchester
Energy	16–44	8.6	7.6	12.4	8.3
	45–64	20.8	10.2	19.4	15.6
	65+	31.8	22.2	32.9	27.6
	all 16+	15.9	11.1	17.9	14.5
Pain	16–44	3.6	1.3	3.2	2.8
	45–64	12.6	3.4	8.0	6.4
	65+	14.8	14.0	16.8	12.9
	all 16+	8.0	4.3	6.9	6.1
Emotional Reactions	16–44	11.4	5.0	11.6	7.6
	45–64	15.9	8.5	14.2	9.6
	65+	17.5	10.1	16.8	12.5
	all 16+	13.7	7.1	13.2	9.2
Sleep	16–44	11.5	8.9	11.8	7.3
	45–64	20.6	14.8	19.3	14.6
	65+	30.0	32.3	26.6	27.8
	all 16+	17.6	15.1	16.5	14.0
Social Isolation	16–44	5.5	1.7	5.0	3.0
	45–64	10.8	5.5	7.1	5.3
	65+	15.2	13.4	11.2	9.4
	all 16+	8.6	5.1	6.7	5.1
Physical Mobility	16–44	2.2	0.9	2.1	1.7
	45–64	9.9	4.0	6.2	5.0
	65+	23.7	20.4	20.5	16.8
	all 16+	7.8	5.5	6.6	5.9

statistically significant differences. Allowing for the fact that the over 64's could not be coded on social class or nationality, the number of statistically significant associations between NHP scores and the social factors measured increased with age.

Curtis rather tentatively concluded from the study that there was some evidence for differences in patterns of morbidity as reported by adults in the boroughs of Tower Hamlets and Redbridge. These differences were most reliable when measured by the NHP, which was the measure least open to variable interpretation and interviewer effects. She further surmised that the differences might have resulted from the different social characteristics of the two communities. However, demographic and social factors interact in a complex way which cannot be thoroughly explored in a large population study such as this.

This impressive and informative piece of research has shown the value of a well established measure of perceived health - in this case the NHP - as a tool for use in population studies. It also provides the reader for the first time with an example of the NHP being used as part of a population study rather than as the focus of the study itself.

The Perceived Health of Unemployed and Employed Workers

This section describes studies comparing and contrasting the perceived health of men in and out of employment. While varying considerably in the size and nature of the samples studied, these studies show the heuristic value of the NHP as a research tool.

Long Term Unemployment and Re-employment.

Much attention has been paid recently to the association between employment status and health. A wide variety of methodologies have been employed to study the association. These have ranged from correlational studies relating levels of unemployment to general health trends in society (see Brenner and Mooney, op cit) to the association between health and employment status at the individual level (see Warr, 1984) some studies relying on only a single item measure of response to unemployment (for example, Feather and Davenport,

Table 6.6: Demographic Variables influencing Scores on Sections of the NHP Data from Curtis's Study of Inner- and outer-London Boroughs: (* = $p < 0.05$).

Age Group	16 – 44						45 – 64						65 and over					
NHP Section	EN	P	EM	SL	SO	PM	EN	P	EM	SL	SO	PM	EN	P	EM	SL	SO	PM
Variable																		
Marital status		*		*					*		*	*						
Social class		*	*						*	*	*							
Housing tenure			*		*	*		*	*		*	*						
Car ownership					*	*	*	*		*	*	*	*	*		*	*	*
Nationality		*											*	*	*		*	*

1981). Qualitative approaches have also been undertaken which provide rich, descriptive accounts of the experience of job loss, but which do not present empirical evidence of the association between health and employment status (for example, Marsden and Duff, 1975, Seabrook, 1982). Warr (op cit) argues that while these approaches have their value, there is also a need for studies examining relatively large samples of people, through the application of more sophisticated measures of a range of important variables - particularly health.

Brenner and Mooney (op cit) argue the case for studies of specific diagnostic categories of illness covering the span of deleterious health outcomes of unemployment. Such studies would require the use of measures of social and physical functioning. Two dilemmas face social scientists attempting to follow this suggestion. The first is that serious morbidity amongst the working population is relatively rare, requiring large study samples before real differences can be found between employed and unemployed populations. The second problem is variation in times between the stressful life event (unemployment) and the resulting health effects. Bunn (1979) reports that time lags between changes in the rates of ischaemic heart disease, infant mortality and suicide associated with changes in unemployment levels vary from 3 to 6 years in Australia. In contrast, Cobb and Kasl (1977) found that elevation of morbidity risk factors are often higher when people anticipate losing their job than when they have actually lost it. To cope with these problems large scale longitudinal studies would be required - expensive both in time and resources. Further, the larger the sample size, the fewer the resources that can be allocated to each individual studied, limiting investigation of the psychological processes relating employment and health status.

One longitudinal study using measures of perceived health has been carried out, which followed up unemployed men for two years and which compared the impact of unemployment on middle class and working class men (McKenna and Payne, 1984). Details of the method by which the original sample was drawn can be found in Payne, Warr and Hartley (1984). Two groups of men who had been unemployed between six and twelve months were selected. They were all married, white and aged between 25 and 39 years. The middle class group was selected from social classes I, II and III n (n=203) and the working class from social classes IV and V (n=196).

The social classification was based on job immediately prior to unemployment. The data presented
here are based on a second wave of interviews with
the same sample - one year after the initial
interview. Men who had regained employment were
also re-interviewed. Attrition of the sample left
146 middle class and 140 working class men.

As part of the study, respondents were asked to
complete the General Health Questionnaire (GHQ) a
self-administered screening test designed to detect
non-psychotic psychiatric disorders (Goldberg,
1972). The 12 item version was used as a measure of
general psychological distress and was supplemented
by 11 other items enabling the calculation of
anxiety and depression subscales (Goldberg and
Hillier, 1979) each of which contained 7 items.
Interviewees were also given a copy of the NHP and a
reply-paid envelope. The completion of the NHP was
optional but 64.7 per cent of the sample returned
usable Profiles. Analysis of responses to the first
interview showed few differences between NHP
responders and non-responders - none of which were
related to health.

Table 6.7: The Perceived Health of Unemployed and
Re-employed Men: Mean Scores on the NHP and GHQ.

Health measure	Unemployed (n=114)	Re-employed (n=71)
Energy	19.30	8.77
Pain	3.29	1.14
Emotional reactions	33.37	7.68
Sleep	27.57	7.63
Social isolation	15.47	3.04
Physical mobility	2.63	0.15
GHQ12	15.67	7.84
Depression	4.13	0.72
Anxiety	8.89	4.42

Table 6.7 shows the mean scores on the NHP and GHQ
for unemployed and re-employed men. All variables
showed statistically significant differences

(p < 0.01), except for pain, where relatively low
scores were obtained from both groups. However, it
should be noted that the re-employed group contained
a greater proportion of middle class respondents.
However, Payne et al (op cit) showed that amongst
the medium term unemployed there were no differences
in GHQ scores by social class. Of the 18 scores
shown in Table 6.7 only one statisically significant
difference (p < 0.05) was found between the social
classes. This was for emotional reactions, where
the mean score for the unemployed middle class men
(24.05) was lower than that for the unemployed
working class men (39.01).

What was perhaps most surprising (and of
interest) was that there were no differences between
the scores of working and middle class respondents
who had regained employment. One can only speculate
how long it would take the social class differences
to reappear, or whether they ever would for people
who had experienced long-term unemployment.
Comparisons can also be made between scores on the
NHP and the norms obtained from the studies
described above. The norms were weighted to match
the age and social class structure of the unemployed
and re-employed samples. These norms are shown in
Table 6.8 together with the mean scores for the two
study populations. It is clear that for all
sections of the NHP the unemployed group scored
significantly higher than the norm, while those who
had become re-employed scored signficantly lower
than the norm on the emotional reactions, social
isolation and physical mobility sections.

Unfortunately, no adequate norms were available
for comparison with the GHQ scores obtained in the
study.

A third round of interviews a year later has
been carried out with those who were employed at the
second stage. Preliminary results suggest that the
scores on the NHP and GHQ of those who still
remained unemployed (now for between 2½ and 3 years)
varied little from scores a year earlier. Those men
who regained employment (after at least 18 months
unemployment) showed statistically significant
improvements in perceived health as measured by the
NHP and GHQ. In fact their scores were comparable
with those for the re-employed men shown in Table
6.8.

Table 6.8: The Perceived Health of Unemployed and Re-employed Workers: Mean Scores on Sections of the NHP and Norms Weighted for Age and Social Class. (*p < 0.05; **p < 0.01)

NHP Sections	Unemployed		Re-employed	
	Present Study	Weighted Norm	Present Study	Weighted Norm
Energy	19.30	9.86**	8.77	7.69
Pain	3.29	1.46*	1.14	1.78
Emotional reactions	33.37	14.18**	7.68	11.10*
Sleep	27.57	14.32**	7.63	10.66
Social isolation	15.47	8.80**	3.04	5.95**
Physical mobility	2.63	1.61	0.15	1.50**

Lay-off and Early Unemployment. For reasons of practicality, most studies of the association between unemployment and health have concentrated on how people who have been out of work for relatively long periods of time are affected. As was discussed earlier, objective changes in levels of morbidity may lag six years or more behind changes in the level of unemployment. However, over-concentration on the long term unemployed may give an inaccurate picture of the impact of unemployment. It has not been unusual for people to drift in and out of employment as a normal working pattern, particularly in such industries as construction or in regions where there is a seasonal demand for labour. A random sample of unemployed persons at any one point in time will include people unable to work, disabled individuals and others who are 'between jobs', as well as a core of the long term unemployed. In recent years this situation has changed somewhat, with in excess of a million people being unemployed for a year or longer.

Consequently, there has been a need to look at how people respond to unemployment in the short term. In particular, it is important to study the effects of recent redundancy on health. In such an area of study measures of perceived health are especially important as morbidity and/or mortality rates will not reflect early health changes - even where unemployment rates may have reached 20 per cent or more of the potential working population.

In order to carry out a study of early unemployment, contact was made with two engineering companies in South Yorkshire. One, Factory A, was embarking on a programme of rotating lay-offs - each for a fixed period of seven weeks and the other, Factory B, was closing down and making its workforce redundant. At Factory A, interviews were conducted with 39 workers on three occasions - before lay-off, in the fifth week of lay-off and finally on return to full-time working. At Factory B it was only possible to interview 20 people in the fifth week following redundancy. This limitation was caused by the company's decision to dismiss a majority of its workers prior to the notified date of redundancy. The study was designed to investigate Jahoda's theory of the latent functions of work (Jahoda, 1981) and to look at changes in perceived health. This discussion will cover only the impact on health as reported by McKenna and Fryer (1984). Readers interested in the other aspects of the study are referred to Fryer and McKenna (1984).

Table 6.9 shows the scores obtained on the NHP for Factory B (interviewed at Time 2 only) and for Factory A on the three administrations of the Profile For comparison, the weighted norm for a working population (see above) is also shown.

It is clear from the table that the redundant workers at Factory B score considerably higher than the norm - but the small population size at the factory plus the high variability of scores on the NHP prevent the difference in means from reaching statistical significance. The data for Factory A show a reduction in perceived health problems over time, except in the sleep section. This section is also unusual in that scores prior to lay-off for sleep problems were significantly lower than those obtained from a normal population. For the pain and physical mobility sections, scores were significantly lower than the norm during and after lay off. Scores on the energy and emotional reactions sections, while showing a gradual improvement over time, were only significantly better than the norm when the respondents were back at work (Time 3). A similar downward trend was found for social isolation but the scores did not differ significantly from the norm on any of the three occasions. Again, because of the small sample sizes, differences in the mean scores between the two factories (at Time 2) were not statistically significant although markedly different in size.

The data for Factory A were subjected to a Friedman two-way analysis of variance to see whether the downward trend in scores on the separate sections was statistically significant. All tests were negative. Closer inspection of the data showed that there were three distinct responses to the lay-off.

Of the 37 respondents who provided three satisfactorily completed Profiles, 9 (24 per cent) had scores which increased at Time 2 and then reduced again on return to work. Sixteen subjects (43 per cent) had scores which improved during lay-off and then returned to the Time 1 levels on return to work. Eight subjects (22 per cent) had scores which were lower at Time 2 and lower again at Time 3. Thus individual workers had differing reactions to their lay-off as measured by the NHP. Qualitative data from the interviews helped explain these different reactions. Those individuals whose perceived health improved during lay-off had planned carefully for the time away from their employment - both financially and in the way in which they were going to use their time. Many respondents found that they spent longer working in a week than when employed. They also valued the freedom of choosing when to work, when to rest and when to take a holiday. In contrast, those workers whose NHP scores increased during lay-off, tended to have prepared less well and to be relatively inactive.

Of course, while the laid-off workers did not see the period as an extended holiday, they did have a finite period over which they would be 'unemployed'. This was not the case for the redundant workers at Factory B. Because they were unable to guess how long they would be without employment, they were less able to plan their time and resources and consequently tended to be less active in terms of carrying out jobs in the home or taking part in sports and leisure activities. Although they were financially better off than the workers from Factory A (having received lump sum redundancy payments) they were unable to judge how long they would have to survive on this amount,

Table 6.9: Mean Scores on Sections of the NHP for Workers from Factories A and B and the Significance of Differences in these Means from those of a Normal Working Population. (*p < 0.05; **p < 0.01).

Section of NHP	Norm for working population matched for age and social class	Factory A Time 1	Factory A Time 2	Factory A Time 3	Factory B
Energy	7.38	13.72	6.59	2.24**	15.12
Pain	3.94	3.65	1.80*	1.99*	9.40
Emotional reactions	8.86	11.51	8.84	4.49**	19.92
Sleep	10.71	6.10	8.80	5.86	23.29
Social isolation	2.96	4.10	3.52	1.53	4.18
Physical mobility	2.27	1.46	0.57**	0.59**	5.91

although many of them used part of the sum to pay off debts or to buy consumer goods which they were renting while employed. This had the added advantage of lowering their savings below the threshold at which supplementary benefits could be claimed.

Similar trends were found for the General Health Questionnaire, which was also completed by respondents. Weighted norms for this 30 item form of the GHQ were derived from a study of unemployed workers by Jackson and Warr (1984). Surprisingly, at Time 2, the scores on the GHQ were significantly lower than the norm for workers from both factories.

These studies of unemployment have shown that measures of perceived health, particularly the NHP, are important tools in the evaluation of the impact of job loss - both in the short- and long-term. What has not been established is whether short-term changes in perceived health ultimately lead to later morbidity. However, scores on the GHQ and NHP have been shown to be highly correlated with overall rated health and reported disease (see for example, Payne et al, op cit). Such questions could only adequately be answered by large scale longitudinal studies of the unemployed using both subjective health measures and clinical assessments of health status.

PROBLEMS ASSOCIATED WITH COMMUNITY STUDIES

Many of the problems associated with carrying out successful population studies are those that attend on all social research. However, in many ways the social scientist has certain advantages. What the traditional scientist may gain in specificity and control over confounding variables, may be lost in the generality of the findings. The immunologist can learn a great deal about the functioning of a single cell - but place that cell in a human body and a completely different set of circumstances apply.

In contrast, the social scientist studies the whole individual or groups of individuals and hopes to learn something from the generality. Within the individual there are many variables over which the researcher has no influence and which he or she is unable to measure or allow for. When a population is under study even more variables will become part of the error variance and will reduce the likelihood of establishing the true influence of those factors which are under study. One crumb of comfort for the researcher is that should a variable be shown to have a predicted effect then he or she can be confident that the 'statistically significant' difference will also be a meaningful one (assuming that an unrealistically large sample size has not been employed).

Asking questions of people is not easy, requiring considerable expertise and experience. The researcher and respondent immediately enter a well rehearsed social activity - that of discussion and seeking another person's views. The respondent may like or dislike the questioner and may be bored or interested in the subject of discussion. Respondents may try to help or hinder the researcher or to avoid saying things which may reflect badly on themselves. The interviewer will also react differently to different respondents - non-verbal signals may be passed which will affect the response.

There is no room here to discuss the problems of interviews and the biases introduced by both the researcher and respondent. Readers interested in pursuing these areas should consult any of the standard texts on experimental design or educational research.

Collecting information by questionnaire overcomes some of these problems but introduces others. No rapport can be built up between respondent and researcher, no check can be made on the accuracy of responses and it is very easy just to ignore unsolicited requests for personal information which arrive in the mail. Despite these problems, interviews and questionnaires are the most useful tools available to the social scientist and every effort must be made to put them to best use.

Sample Size and Sampling

In an ideal world the researcher will determine the necessary sample size by noting the number of variables, estimating the size of effect and the likely error in measurement. Too often one is limited by the number of respondents available or the time and expense involved in surveying sufficient numbers of subjects. Similarly, ideal sampling methods will often be limited by problems of access or the need to avoid costly travel and numerous call-backs to missed appointments. Moser and Kalton (1971) consider sampling theory in terms of urns containing balls of different colours which can be drawn at random. They suggest that the social scientist has to sample from an urn in which some of the balls properly belonging to it happen not to be present at the time of selection, while others obstinately refuse to be taken from it! This is not quite the random sampling of textbooks.

Non-response

There is no way in which population studies can avoid the problems of non-response. However well-designed the study and whatever measures are taken to reduce non-response, some part of the sample will be missed. Of course, if non-response were random, the phenomenon would present no problems. Unfortunately, the missing part of the sample often does differ significantly from the rest. If one considers a study of the health of a population in which people are contacted in their homes, it is clear that no individuals currently in hospital will be included, leading to an underestimate of the ill health in the community. At the same time, those people away from home taking part in sporting activities or who have a busy social life (that is people who are more likely to be 'healthy') may also be missed, leading to an over-estimate of the level of ill health in the community. It is also clear that strenuous attempts to contact the latter non-responders might lead to an even greater bias unless attempts were also made to contact the respondents currently in hospital.

In the average interview survey the non-response rate is likely to be between 10 and 25 per cent, dependent on the nature of the study and the demands made on respondents. Response rates from mailed questionnaire studies are likely to be even lower.

The evidence also shows that non-responders do differ from responders. Lydal (1955) analysed response rates to a National Savings Survey by rateable value of dwelling and size of town. The response rates varied from 84 per cent for a rateable value below £10 to only 51 per cent for a rateable value of £50 and over. For conurbations the response rate was 66 per cent, for other urban towns 77 per cent and for rural towns 86 per cent.

Substitution is generally not a solution to the problem as non-responders are simply replaced by responders. However, where stratified sampling has been employed, substitutes can be made to maintain the planned proportions.

Efforts can be made to reduce the number of non-responders. The first should be to minimise refusals. This can be done by keeping questionnaires brief, easily completable and relevant. Durbin and Stuart (1951) found that experienced professional interviewers had 3 to 4 per cent refusals compared with the 13 per cent of inexperienced amateurs. The refusal rate on a questionnaire study of the then topical subject of tuberculosis was 4 per cent - but double that for questionnaire surveys of reading habits and saving. Our experience is that telephoning to make appointments is a good method of reducing refusals, although it is harder to refuse an interviewer face to face than over the telephone or by letter.

Where prior arrangements to meet by appointment are impossible, recalls should be made where there has been no contact. Edwards (1953) in a study of newspaper readership, had a response rate of 40 per cent after the initial visit rising to 77 per cent on first recall, 93 per cent in second recall and 100 per cent in 8 calls. Clearly it is impractical to make more than 2 or 3 recalls. In the case of questionnaire studies, reminders and sending a second questionnaire also increase response rate, possibly by as much as 50 per cent.

It is possible to correct for non-response by gaining as much information as feasible about the sub-sample of non-respondents. This data should include such details as sex, age, social grouping, type of housing and size of family. The composition of the sample of responders should be compared with known population data, for example, as collected by the most recent census. Where the two samples are similar, the researcher can suppose that the study population is comparable with the population it is taken from - but there is no guarantee that bias does not exist.

In certain cases, where significant differences are found between the sample and the whole population, it is sensible to correct the data by re-weighting the responses. However, where differences in response associated with gender, age grouping or social class are under study, it would be unnecessary to weight the overall scores by these variables. Despite this, varying response rates between, for example, men and women, might well be indicative of bias.

The extent to which one tries to overcome non-response is determined by the nature of the study.

Some attempt at following up non-responders must be made but various economies should be considered. Moser and Kalton (op cit) suggest that it is not essential to go out for complete information from follow-up contacts - a few key items may be sufficient. Researchers can also concentrate on following up non-responders in some carefully selected areas only and use this information to correct the results for the entire sample.

As was touched on above, questionnaire surveys can have lower response rates than interviews - even as low as 10 per cent, although the Government Social Survey has achieved response rates in the region of 90 per cent (Scott, 1961). Scott has shown the importance of the questionnaire's sponsor. Thus, it is commonly found that questionnaires asking about perceived health will achieve a higher response if accompanied by a letter from the individual's general practitioner requesting co-operation in the study.

The nature of the sample population will also influence response. It has been found that the less educated, those from lower social classes and those lacking an interest in the topic have above average non-response. While these findings are not surprising, they may well influence the results of the study considerably. Piloting is important; to determine any obvious causes of non-response, to check the clarity of instructions and explanations and to test the different approaches to gaining the co-operation of respondents - such as different questionnaire formats and covering letters.

The covering letter should make it clear who is collecting the information, how the respondent has been selected and why a response is important. Confidentiality or anonymity should be promised where appropriate. Wherever possible personalised covering letters should be used with the respondent's name on and a personalised signature from the sender. The increasing availability of word processors is a great boon to the researcher carrying out a postal survey. Reply-paid addressed envelopes must be included, as it is unreasonable to expect respondents to pay for the dubious privilege of filling in a form for the benefit of some stranger.

In questionnaire surveys the most effective method of raising the response rate is the use of follow-ups. These are most effective when the same package is sent out with a short covering letter reiterating the importance of responding. The need to send a second questionnaire and reply-paid envelope for return is due to the likelihood that the original package will have been mislaid or thrown away. When follow-up packages are to be sent out, the original questionnaire will have had to have been clearly numbered so that non-respondents can be identified. Certain 'techniques' have been used by researchers to identify responders - such as writing a code number under the stamp on the reply envelope - but such methods are unethical and likely to lead to serious problems if discovered. A far better method is to promise confidentiality rather than anonymity and to explain why it is necessary to have a code number. The 'threat' of a second contact might even increase the response rate. In any case, it seems likely that anonymity is not necessarily preferential to confidentiality in encouraging people to respond.

Moser and Kalton (op cit) suggest that the same proportion of persons sent questionnaires will respond to each mailing. Thus if the initial response rate were 80 per cent, one might expect 80 per cent of the remaining 20 per cent of non-responders to reply to a follow-up (i.e. a further 16 per cent, raising the overall response rate to 96 per cent). As is the case with interviewing, it is possible to follow up only a sub-section of the non-responders and weight the whole sample accordingly. However, mailed questionnaires are relatively cheap to administer and at least two follow-ups to all non-responders could well be worthwhile.

It is also possible to interview a sample of non-responders either directly or by telephone - but there remains the possibility that information collected in this way may differ from that given less personally in the questionnaire.

The likelihood of bias due to low response to questionnaires is very high and every effort should be made to maximise the response rate. Attention to details at an early stage is well worth the effort in terms of response rate and the accuracy of answers given.

Accuracy
The accuracy of responses to interviews and questionnaires again depends on how well the tools have been designed and the nature of the information required. Clearly, it is easier to answer questions about how one feels at the moment than about how one felt in the past or about topics of which one has

little experience. Problems of social acceptability may influence responses to certain questions, for example, about social class or tobacco and alcohol consumption - especially during interview. A further problem can occur where a respondent is unwilling to give information or has some reason to mislead the researchers. It is not uncommon for three different political parties to conduct polls in a single constituency and find that they are all going to win the seat! However, what is perhaps surprising is that people are generally so helpful in providing information and making researchers welcome in their homes.

DISTRIBUTION OF SCORES ON THE NOTTINGHAM HEALTH PROFILE

As has been described in earlier chapters and is clear from the studies reported in this one, scores obtained on the NHP are generally low. Except in populations where there is severe morbidity, a majority of respondents will score zero on one or more sections of Part I and on the whole of Part II. Combining data from the two boroughs studied by Curtis (op cit) the following percentages of respondents scored zero on the six sections of Part I:

Pain	- 83%
Social isolation	- 82%
Physical mobility	- 78%
Energy	- 75%
Emotional reactions	- 61%
Sleep	- 56%

The NHP is clearly tapping only the extreme end of perceived health problems. Such a distribution of responses was built into the NHP during its development. At an early stage it was decided that it would be undesirable to include health problems which would be affirmed by a large proportion of the population. As the Dunnel and Cartwright (1972) survey showed, the experience of symptoms is very common and there was an inverse relationship between the presence of certain symptoms and rated health, with the healthy people having headaches, skin troubles, accidental injuries, trouble with teeth and gums and feet problems more frequently than people who rated their health poor. The most commonly experienced symptoms were headache (38 per cent), coughs, catarrh or phlegm (32 per cent), aches or pains in joints and muscles (29 per cent), backache (21 per cent) and nerves, depression or irritability (21 per cent). Clearly, items in a health profile which related to such relatively trivial morbidity would not be able to discriminate adequately between people with varying health statuses.

By limiting items to relatively severe health problems, responses to the NHP are bound to be skewed towards zero or low scores. This can be illustrated by using Dunnell and Cartwright's data. Figure 6.1 shows the percentage of their population of 1,401 adults who rated their recent health as excellent, good, fair or poor.

From the Figure it would appear that perceived health, as measured on the 4 point scale, approximates to a normal distribution with the mean at or close to 'Good'. The regression line for the mean number of symptoms experienced is also shown. If one were to assume that the NHP detects only problems associated with 'fair' or 'poor' perceived health then only individuals to the right of the vertical line drawn on the Figure would obtain positive scores. If this were the case - that the NHP measures only problems at one extreme of the distribution of perceived health - then it would not be surprising that a majority of respondents score zero.

The implications of such a skewed distribution of scores on the NHP are important because scores obtained are subject to a marked basement effect. Scores of zero on the sections are not indicative of a complete lack of perceived health problems in that domain or of perfect health. It would be possible to have a deteriorating health status which could not be detected by the NHP. For example, as we have just seen the NHP may only detect problems (ie score above zero) when a person's perceived health is 'fair' or 'poor'. On Dunnell and Cartwright's 4 point scale it would be possible for someone to rate his or her health excellent on one occasion and good on a second. This would represent a deterioration in health status but would not lead to a change in score on the NHP - as it would still be zero. Similarly, it would not be possible to interpret a change in score on the Profile from zero to a positive score, except to say that there had been a deterioration in perceived health. With such a distribution, some doubt must be cast on the level of measurement achieved by test scores, i.e. it must

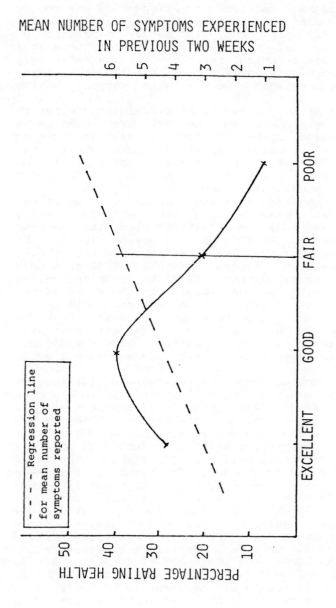

FIGURE 6.1: POPULATION RATED HEALTH AND NUMBER OF SYMPTOMS EXPERIENCED IN PREVIOUS TWO WEEKS. (DATA FROM DUNNEL AND CARTWRIGHT, 1972).

156

be considered that NHP scores form an ordinal or interval rather than a ratio scale.

In chapter 5 it was suggested that scores on the NHP might approximate to a ratio scale, when a rational zero point could be calculated. However, the rational zero derived from regressing scale values had a negative score, i.e. corresponding to some point well to the left of the horizontal axis on Figure 6.1, indicating good or excellent health. As we have seen, the NHP is not able to measure positive perceived health - only perceived health problems - and for almost any population studied the scores will be skewed to the right, with a large proportion scoring zero.

Such distributions of scores can cause problems where statistical analyses are used to compare two populations on more than one occasion. The first modern statistical techniques of inference (parametric techniques) made a number of assumptions about the nature of the population from which the scores were drawn. Two of these assumptions are that the scores are drawn from a population that is normally distributed and that any two or more sets of scores being compared have similar variance or spread (as measured by the standard deviation).

When dealing with scores on the NHP it is possible that either or both of these assumptions are not achieved. In theory this would invalidate the use of parametric statistical techniques, although some statisticians would argue that the assumptions need not necessarily apply, particularly for such robust tests as the ubiquitous t-test.

More recently a large number of techniques of inference have been developed which do not make numerous or stringent assumptions about 'parameters' (population values). These newer - nonparametric ('distribution-free') - techniques do not depend on the shape of the population from which the scores are drawn. These techniques are sometimes referred to as 'ranking tests' and focus on the order or ranking of the scores, not on their 'numerical' values. The nonparametric tests can be almost as powerful as parametric tests in detecting real differences between two sets of scores, especially when there are large sample sizes, and the researcher may well decide that it is more appropriate to employ nonparametric statistical techniques. Siegel (1956) provides a comprehensive and readily understandable description of non-parametric tests.

One advantage of the ranking methods is that

they do not give undue influence to scores obtained from individuals who have abnormally high scores. This is of particular importance with small samples, as the following example will show. Let us assume that we are comparing the scores of two groups of patients on the emotional reactions section of the NHP. It should be remembered that scores can range from zero to 100 with a higher score indicating greater perceived health problems. Table 6.10 shows the hypothetical scores obtained.

In group A, 4 individuals scored zero and 4 had positive scores, one scoring the maximum 100, indicating the presence of all the emotional reactions problems. The mean NHP score for group A was 20.6. In group B, 3 individuals scored zero and five had positive scores, although the highest was only 25. The mean score for this group was 7.8. Thus the mean scores for the two groups differ considerably, mainly due to the subjects in group A who scored 50 and 100 respectively. Table 6.10 also shows the combined ranks and mean ranks for each group.

The combined ranks are calculated by listing the scores from both groups together from lowest to highest (or vice versa) as follows:

0,0,0,0,0,0,0,3,5,6,10,20,25,50,100.

These scores are then ranked from 1 to 16 (as there are 16 subjects in the combined sample). Where scores are tied the mean rank is allocated to each subject with the same score. Hence the rank for a score of zero is $[(1+2+3+4+5+6+7)/7] = 4$.

As can be seen from Table 6.10 the mean ranks for the two groups are identical. Parametric techniques would compare the two group means, while nonparametric techniques would be concerned with the difference between the mean ranks. The latter type of analysis minimises the effect of extreme scores which have an undue influence on means. It is not unusual when studying groups of subjects to find some individuals with abnormally high scores on the NHP who, especially where the population sizes are small, would probably distort the mean perceived health score for the whole group. Where this is likely to occur nonparametric techniques should be employed. With larger population samples, the influence of these 'outliers' on the mean will be less marked and the use of parametric techniques might be considered.

Table 6.10: Hypothetical Scores and combined Rank Value obtained on the Emotional Reactions Section of the NHP by Two Groups of Respondents.

Group A scores	Combined rank value for each Group A score	Group B scores	Combined rank value for each Group B score
0	4	0	4
0	4	0	4
0	4	0	4
0	4	3	8
5	9	6	10
10	12	7	11
50	15	20	13
100	16	25	14
Mean 20.6	8.5	7.8	8.5

CONCLUSIONS

The final section of this chapter has looked at some of the issues which should concern people using the NHP as a research tool. Every effort should be made to select the population carefully and to minimise non-response, in order to avoid biasing the data collected. Such issues of sampling have import for all population studies using any form of data collection.

Problems of concern specifically to the NHP are the distribution of scores obtained which will, in almost every study, be highly skewed. Where this occurs, careful consideration should be given to the statistical tests used to analyse the data collected. Many studies have been undertaken where doubts about the methods of statistical analysis arise and many instruments are employed in population studies which fail to meet the criteria for parametrical analysis (although they may appear to do so).

REFERENCES

Brenner, M.H. and Mooney, A. (1983) 'Unemployment and Health in the Context of Economic Change', Soc Sci Med, 17, 1125-1138

Cobb, S. and Kasl, S.V. (1977) The Consequences of Job Loss, NIOSH, Research Report No. 77-224 US Department of Health, Education and Welfare Washington DC

Curtis, S. (1985) Intra-Urban Variations in Health Care, Volume 1, Department of Geography and Earth Science, Queen Mary College, London University, London

Dunnell, K. and Cartwright, A. (1972) Medicine Takers, Prescribers and Hoarders, Routledge and Kegan Paul, London

Durbin, J. and Stuart, A. (1951) 'Differences in Response Rates of Experienced and Inexperienced Interviewers', J Roy Stat Soc, A, 117, 387-428

Edwards, F. (1953) 'Aspects of Random Sampling for a Commercial Survey', Incorporated Statistician, 4, 9-26

Feather, N.T. and Davenport, P.R. (1981) 'Unemployment and Depressive Affect: A Motivational Analysis', J Pers Soc Psychol, 41, 422-436

Fryer, D. and McKenna, S.P. (1984) 'An Investigation of the Impact of Lay-off and Redundancy on Well Being and the Latent Functions of Employment',

MRC/ESRC Social and Applied Psychology Unit Sheffield University, Sheffield

Goldberg, D.P. (1972) The Detection of Psychiatric Illness by Questionnaire, Oxford University Press, London

Goldberg, D.P. and Hillier, V.F. (1979) 'A Scaled Version of the General Health Questionnaire', Psychol Med, 9, 1339-145

Goldthorpe, J. and Llewellyn, C. (1977) 'Class Mobility: Intergenerational and Work Life Patterns', Brit J Sociol, 28, 269-302

Her Majesty's Stationery Office, (1974) 1971 Census, England and Wales, General Tables, HMSO, London

Hunt, S.M. McEwen, J. and McKenna, S.P. (1985) 'Social Inequalities and Perceived Health', Effective Health Care, 2, 151-160

Jackson, P.R. and Warr, P.B. (in press) 'Unemployment and Psychological Ill Health: The Moderating Role of Duration and Age', Psychol Med

Jahoda, M. (1981) 'Work, Employment and Unemployment' Amer Psychol, 36, 184-191

Leavey, R. (1982) Inequalities in Urban Primary Care Use and Acceptability of G.P. Services, DHSS Research Unit, Dept. of General Practice, University of Manchester, Manchester

Lydall, H.F. (1955) British Incomes and Savings, Oxford University Institute of Statistics Monograph No. 5, Blackwell, Oxford

McEwen, J. Lowe, D. Hunt, S.M. and McKenna, S.P. (1985) 'The Workplace: An Opportunity to Promote Health based on the Measurement of Perceived Health?', Unpublished report, Dept of Community Medicine, King's College School of Medicine and Dentistry, London

McKenna, S.P. and Payne, R.L. (1984) 'A Comparison of the General Health Questionnaire and the Nottingham Health Profile in a Study of Unemployed and Re-employed Men', MRC/ESRC Social and Applied Psychology Unit, University of Sheffield, Sheffield

Marsden, D. and Duff, E. (1975) Workless: Some Unemployed Men and their Families, Penguin, Harmondsworth

Moser, C.A. and Kalton, G. (1971) Survey Methods in Social Investigation, (2nd ed), Heinemann, London

Office of Population Censuses and Surveys (1970) Classification of Occupations, HMSO, London

Office of Population Censuses and Surveys (1983) General Household Survey 1981, Series GHS, No. 11 HMSO, London

Payne, R.L. Warr, P.B. and Hartley, J. (1984) 'Social Class and Psychological Ill-Health during Unemployment', Sociol Hlth Illness, 6, 152-174

Perkins, E. (1984) Health Education in the Work-place. Guidelines for Action, Health Education, Council, London

Scott, C. (1961) 'Research on Mail Surveys' J Roy Stat Society, A, 124, 143-205

Seabrook, J. (1982) Unemployment, Quartet Books, London

Siegel, S. (1956) Nonparametric Statistics for the Behavioural Sciences, McGraw-Hill, Kogakusha, London

Vernon, P.E. (1960) Intelligence and Attainment Tests, University of London Press Ltd, London

Warr, P.B. (1984) 'Economic Recession and Mental Health: A Review of Research', Tijdschrift Voor Sociale Gezondheidszorg, 62, 298-309

Chapter 7.

HEALTH INDICATORS IN CLINICAL CARE

As we have seen in previous chapters, the commonest reason for seeking health care is 'not feeling well' and most patients would hope that as a result of care, treatment or advice, they will 'feel better'. Such changes in feelings may be produced by the specific treatment of a diagnosed disease or injury, by symptomatic treatment designed to reduce the impact of a disease, whether or not diagnosed, by the normal recovery mechanisms within the body or by an improvement resulting from personal support, group discussion, information and education, self-care or environmental change. Whatever the type and level of intervention, the patient is able to form some assessment of the value of the care, through the change or lack of change in self-perceived health.

The efficacy and effectiveness of medical or surgical procedures are normally based upon clinical tests and doctors' assessments using a number of parameters appropriate to the particular problem, but increasingly in scientific papers on treatment there is a reference to 'quality of life'. In life-threatening cases, outcome has usually been measured by survival rates and in less severe conditions by some assessment of disability. Patients' views on their own health are often sought by doctors during consultations, but frequently, as we have seen, there is a lack of agreement between doctor and patients on the outcome of care. Sometimes such discrepancies are the result of a failure by doctors to explain the purpose of care which may not be aimed at improving the patient's feelings of health, but more often they are due to different inter-pretations of outcome based on different concerns.

Indicators such as the Nottingham Health Profile have a potential role in clinical care which may be of value to both patients and health professionals in a variety of areas of clinical practice. The use of the Profile in this setting is relatively new and few studies are yet complete. Most are preliminary investigations rather than carefully and rigorously designed studies. It is hoped that these preliminary ideas will encourage those planning clinical studies to consider the Nottingham Health Profile as an aid to the assessment of outcome.

DECIDING ON TREATMENT

A strange dilemma between medical practice and personal feelings seems to affect both patients and professionals as to the basis for choice of treatment. On one hand, the emphasis is on the rational scientific evidence that a particular drug has proven ability to intervene in the disease process, while on the other hand, attention is paid to the choice of drug to suit the individual patient. Patients often give accounts of the many drugs that a doctor tried before the 'right' one was found. Advertisements for drugs may present the same, dual approach. 'Compared with standard therapy, 'X' has a highly specific and more physiological approach to treatment' and 'After all, no-one wants to feel under the weather when they could be feeling good'. What is, or should be, the basis for deciding on the best treatment?

It is one of the commonest claims of the medical profession that good therapeutic decisions arise from years of clinical experience and this clinical feedom is guarded jealously by doctors. However, it is also recognised that there should be a rational basis relating to the best available evidence underlying such clinical experience and this is being taught increasingly in medical schools. New forms of medical records are being designed to record the process of relating decisions to evidence. Sackett, Haynes and Tugwell (1985) have analysed the three principal decisions that determine the rational treatment of any patient.

1. Identifying the ultimate objective of treatment. Is the ultimate objective to achieve cure, palliation, symptomatic relief or what?
2. Selecting the specific treatment. Does the patient require any treatment at all?

3. Specifying the treatment target. How will you know when to stop treatment, change its intensity or switch to some other treatment?

What sort of evidence, from what sources, should determine the choice of specific treatment to be used to reach this goal?

The authors consider that these three primary decisions 'when consciously carried out and conscientiously noted in the clinical records can lead to consistent, coherent patient management even when responsibility is shared by several clinicians or a whole team'. However, they go on to point out that:

> ... since any decision about the ultimate objective of treatment is made for the sake of the patient, most clinicians involve, and even defer to, the patient's wishes (or those of an impaired patient's family in this decision). Moreover, when assessing the risks and benefits of specific treatments, the patient's perspectives on their risks and benefits (especially as they involve trade-offs between the quantity and quality of life) may not be only useful but crucial.

There is often an impression in medical literature or in discussions that the importance of considering the patient's perspective is to improve 'compliance'. Doctors are very concerned when patients do not take the medicines prescribed, alter the dosage, or do not complete a defined course of treatment. Literature abounds on the problems of non-compliance and many ways of improving the situation have been suggested. Dunnell and Cartwright (1972) summarised the position on compliance: 2.5 per cent of prescriptions are not followed at all; 16 per cent of the items prescribed are thrown away before being used up and 20 per cent of the medicines are not taken as directed. More recently, studies in general practice or with chronic illness suggest that compliance runs about 50 per cent. It is often recognised that non-compliance may be utterly logical from the patient's perspective; feeling better, the occurrence of unexpected and unexplained side-effects or sometimes the signs of drug toxicity are all good reasons for discontinuing treatment. Solutions to non-compliance tend to be seen in improved doctor-patient communication and education. Conrad (1985) describes the alternative patient-centred approach to managing medications and points out that what appears to be non-compliance from a medical perspective may actually be a form of asserting control over one's own disorder.

This emphasis on mutual decision making would seem to indicate the value of including a shared outcome measure of perceived health as the basis for reviewing therapeutic intervention.

Appropriate outcome measures will have to be determined for each situation. As shown in chapter 4, studies which have compared doctor and patient definition with the outcome of intervention have demonstrated that there is often considerable disagreement, with the doctor focusing attention on wound healing, radiological changes and biochemical tests, while the patient is more concerned with symptoms, loss of function or inability to carry out everyday tasks. As will be shown later in this chapter, the relationship between clinical estimates and measures on the Profile can be examined in properly designed clinical studies and, from such work, an appropriate battery of measures can be used in particular clinical situations with individual patients.

Many clinical conditions as taught to medical students have a distinctive pattern of signs and symptoms. Thyroid disease is an excellent example of this as there may be debate as to which symptoms or signs are necessary for diagnosis or which collection of signs and symptoms are sufficient to indicate the presence of the disease. Some of these relate to general feelings of cold or heat or anxiety while some will have to be sought specifically. An overall measurement of subjective health could provide a general indicator of health status.

Diseases of the thyroid are fairly common, particularly in women: the overall prevalence of goitre may be up to 9 per cent; approximately 2 per cent of women will have an episode of hyper-thyroidism and 1.5 per cent will become hypo-thyroid. Despite the classical descriptions of clinical disease, the diagnosis and management of thyroid disorder now rest considerably, but not solely, on laboratory tests of thyroid function (Himsworth, 1985) and this means that an indication of patients' health would be useful as a linked assessment to these laboratory tests. The following case provides an example of the changes that may

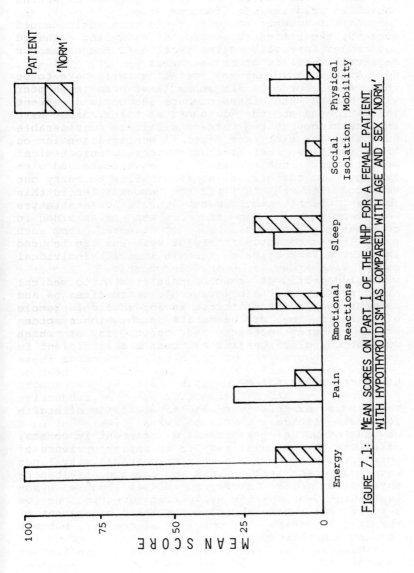

FIGURE 7.1: MEAN SCORES ON PART I OF THE NHP FOR A FEMALE PATIENT WITH HYPOTHYROIDISM AS COMPARED WITH AGE AND SEX 'NORM'

167

take place following treatment.

A previously healthy woman in her early fifties was admitted to hospital with a diagnosis of hypothyroidism. On admission, prior to any treatment, her score on Part I of the NHP was as shown in Figure 7.1. For comparison purposes, the 'norm' for a woman of this age is included. As can be seen, the patient's scores on Energy and Pain are way above average, with Emotional Reactions and Physical Mobility scores somewhat higher. However, her scores on Sleep and Social Isolation are lower than the 'norm'. Six weeks later after treatment with one of the standard drugs she again completed the NHP and scored nil on all sections, indicating that her recovery had been considerably quicker than her slow deterioration prior to hospital admission. At this time, her biochemical tests indicated the satisfactory achievement of replacement hormone therapy. A further six weeks later, she again had no score on the NHP and she verbally indicated a further slight improvement. The fact that she was now scoring well below the norm was probably due to contrast effects.

Thus it would be relatively easy to include the NHP as a routine measure in individual clinical care with results being incorporated into the medical notes. It would be possible to compare the NHP scores with biochemical estimations. The patient would benefit from seeing a visible record of 'feeling better' and this might aid communication between patient and doctor and increase understanding of the aims of treatment.

DIFFERING EXPECTATIONS OF CARE

The above example was of a relatively straight-forward clinical condition with clear cut and obvious symptoms where standard treatment is usually effective and normally results in rapid improvement. However, there are a number of clinical situations which are less well defined and the expectations of care are often different between patient and professional. This is well illustrated in elective surgery for chronic conditions which can be set in the wider debate on what is unnecessary surgery (Schact and Pemberton, 1985).

Usually the patients who undergo such surgery have had a period of disease which produced symptoms or had an obvious swelling or complained of a disfiguring condition. Thus patients are familiar with the impact of their problem on their life and find it relatively easy to make comparisons after the surgical procedure. Usually the procedure is a straightforward and tested operation with a very low risk of mortality and a well recognised time period for healing and recovery. Many surgeons are aware that there is not such a standard view of patient satisfaction. Many studies of different clinical problems show considerable variation in outcome as measured by traditional measures, such as time of return to work, relief from symptoms and general patient satisfaction.

Surgical outpatient clinics in hospital see large numbers of patients who are considered for elective surgery and there is often difficulty in making decisions as to which patients are most likely to benefit from surgery (McColl, Drinkwater, Hulme-Moir and Donnan 1971). Although it is not being considered here, there is also the question as to the best allocation of health service resources.

Hunt, McEwen, McKenna, Backett and Pope (1984) carried out a small study which was designed to compare the perceived health status of patients who underwent surgery with those who remained on the waiting list for a similar period of time. The sample included patients with cysts, polyps, non-malignant swellings, hernias, varicose veins, haemorrhoids and diseased gall bladders.

Patients attending the outpatients' clinic of a General Hospital fell into four categories: a group present for 'clerking' prior to entering the hospital for an operation the following week; patients being followed up after operation; patients on conservative treatment; and new referrals. Patients were approached whilst waiting to see the doctor. If they agreed to take part in the study they were given a copy of the NHP and asked to complete it at home in the next couple of days and to return it in the pre-paid envelope provided. They were told that they would receive another health questionnaire in approximately eight weeks.

Data were collected over a period of four months during the summer. Out of 231 patients approached, 193 returned both questionnaires. Those patients (15) attending for vasectomy operations were considered atypical of the group and were excluded from the analysis. A further 21 subjects were discarded as they returned incomplete questionnaires. The initial scores on Part I and Part II are shown in Table 7.1 and Table 7.2 and are based upon the remaining 157 cases of patients suffering from minor disorders, prior to surgery (i.e. at the time of the first questionnaire).

As can be seen there is quite a high level of perceived health problems with the main problems in the areas of sleep and lack of energy. Some pain and emotional reactivity is present, but there are few problems of physical mobility or social isolation. Daily life is somewhat disrupted mainly in relation to household tasks, sex and holidays but personal relationships are relatively unaffected.

Of these 157 cases, 41 underwent surgery in the week following the return of the first questionnaire. These subjects were allocated to the experimental group. From the remaining 116 cases, a subject was selected who was matched with each experimental subject as closely as possible on the following criteria: age, sex, diagnostic category and date of initial contact in the outpatients department. None of these matched subjects had undergone surgery prior to the completion of the second questionnaire. The matched subjects were used as a quasi-control group for the experimental group. This second group could not be assumed to be closely matched with the experimental group as two patients diagnosed as suffering from a similar complaint might have considerable differences in the severity of their condition, may have had the condition for differing lengths of time and might also differ in other respects such socio-economic status.

Table 7.1: Mean Score on Part I of NHP for Patients attending Out-patient Clinic for Minor Surgical Conditions (n=157).

Energy	24.2
Pain	15.9
Emotional reactions	14.7
Sleep	18.7
Social isolation	5.1
Physical mobility	7.3

The study found that there was very little change in the perceived health status of those undergoing surgery, as shown in Tables 7.3 and 7.4. The experimental and quasi-control groups were

Table 7.2: Percentage of Patients reporting Areas of their Life adversely affected by Health Problems on Part II of the NHP (n=157)

	%
Jobs of work	21.0
Jobs around the house	27.0
Home life	10.8
Social life	27.0
Sex life	24.0
Hobbies and interests	17.8
Holidays	28.7

Table 7.3: Mean Scores on Part I of the NHP of Experimental and Quasi-control Groups before and after Surgical Intervention.

Section	Experimental (n=41)		Control (n=41)	
	Before	After	Before	After
Energy	18.5	16.2	18.7	14.2
Pain	11.9	7.6	13.6	9.7
Emotional reactions	14.7	10.8	13.1	14.7
Sleep	13.2	16.4	18.3	16.4
Social isolation	5.0	5.9	5.4	5.1
Physical mobility	4.5	6.7	8.6	8.4

compared for significant differences in perceived health and areas of life affected at the pre-operational stage and no statistical differences were found. A comparison of the scores of the experimental subjects before and after operation show no significant change on any section of the NHP, nor was there any change in the scores of the quasi-control group. Those who had had an operation were subjectively almost identical to the comparison group who had not undergone surgery. As the study included a variety of disorders, no single explan-ation for these findings is likely to suffice, but several alternatives, which are not mutually excusive, may be suggested.

Table 7.4: Percentage of Patients in Experimental and Quasi-control Groups affirming Statements on Part II before and after Surgical Intervention.

Area	Experimental (n=41)		Control (n=41)	
	Before %	After %	Before %	After %
Occupation	30.0	24.3	24.3	12.2
Jobs around the house	27.5	14.6	22.5	17.0
Personal relationships	12.5	7.3	7.9	4.9
Social life	22.5	19.5	17.1	12.2
Sex life	10.2	17.0	16.6	22.0
Hobbies	27.5	15.0	19.5	19.5
Holidays	22.5	12.5	21.9	12.2

In some instances, procedures may be carried out primarily to prevent complications of existing disease and may not be directed at the treatment of current symptoms. The surgical removal of a gall bladder following early indications of inflammation may be done to prevent more serious disease in later years from gallstones, rather than to relieve vague symptoms of abdominal discomfort.

Different perceptions of recovery time may provide a partial explanation. Although in the opinion of the surgeon, patients should have improved after six weeks on the basis of wound healing and recovery of physiological functioning, feelings of discomfort and tiredness may continue. Thus any improvement in well-being may take longer than the time for wound healing and in the early post-operation period new, temporary, problems associated with the surgical procedure may mask the diminution in pre-operation symptoms.

For some conditions, patients presenting for care may have felt chronically 'under par' from a number of health and social problems and the presenting medical problem may have been largely irrelevant to how they felt. This is supported by the finding that those patients with cysts, ganglions or superficial lumps did not differ significantly from those with the more symptomatic conditions such as hernias, varicose veins or ulcers. Overall health status may, in some cases, be more important in the decision to seek care than is the effect of the actual condition deemed suitable for treatment.

It has been suggested that significant changes in health after medical intervention are experienced only by those who felt relatively unwell before treatment. This has been well documented in accounts of peptic ulcer surgery (Hall, Horrocks, Clamp and Dombal 1976; Cay, Philip, Small, Neilson and Henderson, 1975) and many surgeons are reluctant to operate unless severe symptoms have been present for a considerable period of time.

Other investigations have reported that psychological factors were more important than medical factors in influencing relief from symptoms after operation for peptic ulcer.

To test the hypothesis that improvement is related to levels of ill health prior to surgery, patients were divided into high, medium and low scorers based on their pre-surgery NHP scores, and the data re-analysed. No significant associations between pre-test scores and direction or amount of change were found on Part I of the NHP. On Part II it was found that those patients reporting problems with their social life before surgery were more likely to perceive an overall improvement in Part I after surgery than those with no social problems. Changes in the reported condition of the comparison group over this period of time were also analysed and no significant associations were found.

It is possible that there is a 'threshold' for problems which must be exceeded before patients feel benefit from surgical intervention. Many of this sample had zero or low scores on sections of the NHP and few scores could be regarded as high. It may be, therefore, that health status before the operation was not sufficiently poor for it to be expected to improve significantly, although it should be remembered that a zero score does not indicate perfect health. The patients in this study did not have life threatening or seriously disabling problems, but they do represent a major workload within the health service. As experimental and quasi-control groups did not differ in health status, perceived health alone was unlikely to be the basis for selection for operation and other factors must have influenced patients' and surgeon's choices.

Rather than producing answers, this preliminary study seems to have indicated that longer and larger studies would be beneficial in clarifying the benefits expected and achieved by patients undergoing minor surgery. Similarly, expectations of surgeons and those responsible for planning such surgical services might be more realistic if rigorous data from well designed studies were available.

REVIEWING 'NORMALITY': THE CASE OF PREGNANCY

Although it is important to know more about the effects of disease and disability, it is equally vital to have new insights into something which is regarded as a normal physiological process but which may have a considerable impact on health. An extensive body of literature has documented the physical, social and psychological concomitants of pregnancy, but less is known of the perceptions of health that exist at the different stages of this process.

The first trimester in pregnancy has been described as an 'adaptation' phase, both in physical and in psycho-social terms. Major physiological changes are taking place during the early weeks, with a rapid increase in hormone levels.

Symptoms such as nausea and vomiting and feelings of lethargy are common; increased anxiety and emotional lability are also characteristic of this phase. By about 16 weeks, physiological balance has generally been restored, morning sickness is usually past and a feeling of well-being develops. Over this second trimester, the increasing size of the uterus is liable to cause awkwardness and minor physical discomfort, but women tend to become more tranquil emotionally, slowing down both mentally and physically. Around this time they may start to withdraw from social and work activities (Leifer, 1977).

Over the period of pregnancy many women experience a decline in libido and sexual satisfaction, and this is particularly marked in the third trimester (Lumley, 1978). By this time and especially in the last weeks, the enlarged uterus brings many discomforts - backache, cramps, varicose veins, constipation and shortness of breath are all familiar side effects of later pregnancy. These symptoms tend to be exaggerated at night, leading to disturbed sleep. Anxiety levels are likely to rise again in the last weeks as the delivery becomes imminent (Lubin, Gardener and Roth, 1975).

During pregnancy - particularly a first pregnancy - a number of psycho-social adjustments are required of the woman: acceptance of her changing body image; adjustment to her new role and responsibilities as a mother and consequent readjustment of her relationship with her partner and with her own mother. For the working woman, there will be the need to cope with the financial, social and personal implications of leaving work (Kitzinger, 1972).

For a majority of women, the changes which occur and the adjustments required can be accommodated without major difficulty, and the nine months of pregnancy may be viewed positively as an opportunity for personal and social development. The ease of adaptation to pregnancy is related to the woman's physical, social and emotional well-being. For women with a pre-existing medical condition (such as diabetes or essential hypertension) the older primigravidae, the high gravidity women and those with a history of obstetric or gynaecological problems, pregnancy entails a relatively high risk of complications. Similarly, those who lack emotional or social stability, notably, the very young, the socially disadvantaged and unmarried mothers, are more likely to experience a difficult pregnancy. Complications such as hyperemesis gravidarum, toxaemia and hypertension as well as severe anxiety and depression have been shown to relate to social and psychological pressures. Conversely, one of the best indicators of a successful pregnancy is said to be a stable marriage and a supportive partner (Macy and Faulkner, 1979).

A small study (Williams, Lindsay, Hunt and McKenna, unpublished) based on 80 women who each completed three profiles during a normal pregnancy may help to illustrate the additional information that may be obtained by the use of an instrument like the NHP and how, within a normal pregnancy, there may be considerable variation.

The criteria for inclusion in this study were that the women should be aged between 18 and 35 years, having a first, second or third baby, be free from any chronic conditions existing prior to the pregnancy and likely to lead to complications, be free of any serious physical or mental handicap and have no history of late or repeated miscarriage or neonatal death.

One hundred women were recruited to the study over a six week period. Women who met the specified criteria and were between 12 and 18 weeks of gestation were identified by clinic midwives who then referred them to a member of the research team present at the clinic. Only one woman who was asked to take part in the study declined to do so. Following this personal contact, each subject was sent a copy of the NHP, together with a covering letter and a stamped addressed envelope at 18, 27 and 36 weeks gestation. A total of 20 patients were excluded from the study for the following reasons; they had moved out of the area during the pregnancy; miscarriage; premature birth; admission to hospital with complications; failure to return all the questionnaires and administrative reasons. In addition to completing the NHP subjects were asked to provide an overall assessment of their health on a 5 point scale from 'very good' to 'very bad' and brief details of any medical or social problems.

The median scores of the sample on each section of Part I at 18, 27 and 37 weeks gestation are shown in Figure 7.2. The percentage of women reporting problems in each of the seven areas of daily life are shown in 7.3. A Friedman two-way analysis of variance was carried out on each section to test for significant differences in scores between the three stages of gestation. Statistically significant differences were found in the pain, physical mobility and sleep sections. There was no statistically significant change over time on the social isolation section. Some differences were apparent on energy and emotional reactions but these did not reach statistical significance at the 0.05 level, probably because, although changes were occuring over time these were masked in the analysis by the fact that scores at the first and third stages were similar.

There was considerable variation in the proportion of women experiencing problems on the different sections. For example, only 15-20 per cent of women experienced social isolation problems at any one stage, but 89 per cent of the sample reported problems of physical mobility at 37 weeks.

The relationship between perceived medical and social problems and scores on the NHP was examined. Comparisons were made at each gestation stage

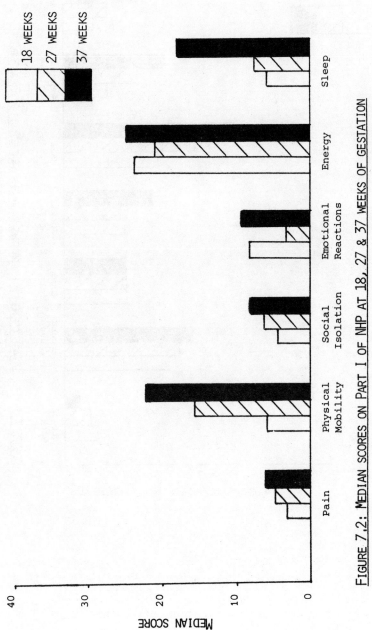

FIGURE 7.2: MEDIAN SCORES ON PART I OF NHP AT 18, 27 & 37 WEEKS OF GESTATION

177

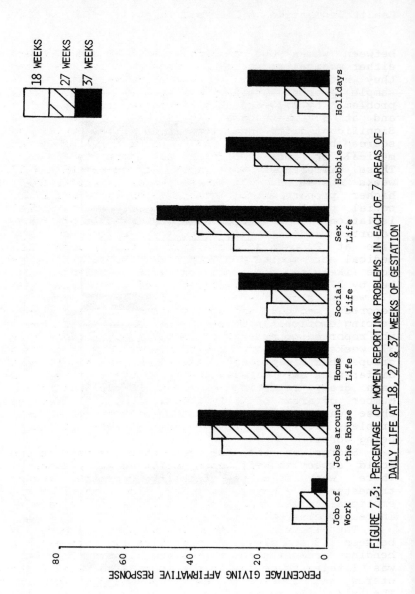

FIGURE 7.3: PERCENTAGE OF WOMEN REPORTING PROBLEMS IN EACH OF 7 AREAS OF DAILY LIFE AT 18, 27 & 37 WEEKS OF GESTATION

178

between women who reported that they had problems
either medical or social and those who reported that
they had none. At 18 weeks, 60 per cent of the
sample reported that they had some medical or social
problem; by 27 weeks this had fallen to 44 per cent
and at 37 weeks the figure was 50 per cent.
Significant differences were found in the pattern of
scores between women who reported that they had
medical or social problems and those who did not.
These differences were most marked at 18 and 27
weeks gestation. At these times a significantly
higher proportion of women reporting medical or
social problems also reported problems of social
isolation, energy and sleep. In addition, women
reported significantly more health effects on their
life at 27 than 18 weeks. At 18 weeks, women with
medical or social problems were also significantly
more likely to report problems of physical mobility,
but by 27 weeks this difference had disappeared. At
27 weeks significantly more women in the group who
reported medical or social problems were experiencing emotional problems, when compared with those
who reported no medical or social complications. By
37 weeks, most of the differences between the two
groups had disappeared. There remained significant
differences only between the proportions of women in
each group reporting sleep problems; and in the
number of areas of daily life affected. In each of
these cases, the group with medical or social
problems again perceived their health status as
being worse.
    Scores on the NHP reflected the pattern one
would expect in well women during normal pregnancy.
There was relative stability over the second
trimester but a marked increase in both physical and
emotional problems by the end of the third, with an
increased disruption in daily life.
    The increase in problems of physical mobility
between 18 and 27 weeks; specifically difficulty in
bending, reaching for things and standing for long,
was likely to be due to the increasing size of the
uterus and consequent awkwardness and discomfort.
The rise in reported sleep disturbance is also
explicable in these terms. The slight fall in
emotional reactions score over this period, though
not statistically significant, is also of interest.
It may have been due to the fact that the first
assessment at 18 weeks, occurred as the women were
emerging from the early 'adjustment' phase; whilst
at 27 weeks their pregnancy would be fully established both physiologically and psychologically

and so a greater degree of emotional stability might
be expected. By the time the third assessment was
made, the women were in the last month of pregnancy,
the phase when problems come to the fore once again.
Physical awkwardness, increasing discomfort, sleep
disturbance and tiredness, as well as mild
depression, are all familiar effects of late
pregnancy, and these were clearly mirrored in the
NHP scores.

Overall, scores were relatively low, no median
score at any stage exceeded 25. This is a
reflection of the fact that the sample chosen
comprised well women who might be expected to
experience a normal pregnancy. The lowest scores
were on the pain section, as might be expected in
such a sample, and those problems which did arise
related mainly to pain at night and finding it painful to change position; both explicable in terms of
the increasing size and weight of the uterus, and
consequent discomforts such as cramp and backache.
Social isolation scores remained consistently low
throughout. Though intuitively some increase might
have been expected, as more women gave up going out
to work, in fact, as the literature indicates,
pregnant women tend to withdraw voluntarily both
socially and psychologically as the pregnancy
progresses; hence feelings of social isolation may
be less likely to arise at this time.

The Nottingham Health Profile was able to
distinguish between women experiencing a 'normal'
pregnancy and those whose pregnancy was complicated
by medical, social or psychological stresses. The
lack of significant difference in the proportion of
women in each group (i.e. women with and without
complicating factors) reporting emotional reactions
at 18 weeks may seem surprising. However, although
emotional problems occurred amongst 55 per cent of
the sample at this stage, there were marked
differences in the severity of the problems reported
by the two groups. The median score on emotional
reactions for women with medical or social problems
was 18.7, compared with a median score of 4.1 for
women with no such problems. A similar situation
occurred with problems of physical mobility at 27
weeks: 69 per cent of the sample reported some
problems at this stage, but the median score for the
group with medical or social problems was approximately twice that of the group without - 21.8
compared with 11.1.

The major differences in the perceived health
of the two groups arose in the second trimester of

pregnancy at 18 and 27 weeks. For well women experiencing normal pregnancy, the second trimester is considered to be the most settled and uneventful, so that a low level of perceived problems on the NHP might be expected. Women experiencing stresses beyond those of normal pregnancy were more likely to have problems. However, by the end of the third trimester, a degree of disruption both physical and emotional, may be considered normal, even for well women - hence the merging of the characteristics of the two groups.

Part II of the NHP reflected the increasing disruption of daily life associated with pregnancy, especially in the areas of sex and looking after the home. As would be expected in this group of women, effects on personal relationships remained about the same over the period of the study.

Although this study was designed to assist with the development of the Nottingham Health Profile, the results may be of value to health professionals by indicating the impact of a 'normal' pregancy and the problems that patients perceive. More extensive studies could be used to inform antenatal education and assist in explaining to those preparing for a pregnancy the changes that are likely to occur throughout the nine months. If profiles were obtained throughout antenatal care, the high scores might serve as an indicator of risk, but further work would be required in both normal and abnormal pregnancies to test the validity of this.

A NEW TREATMENT

Research aimed at the discovery of a new drug or a new therapeutic regimen is one of the most important activities of the pharmaceutical industry and vast resources are devoted to development, testing and marketing. Similarly, staff in medical schools and research institutions are equally committed to developing new equipment or surgical techniques and procedures which will be regarded as a significant advance. Although the financial rewards may be less than with new drugs the resulting prestige or personal status may be an equivalent reward.

After initial work and tests, new approaches are normally submitted to clinical trials before widespread adoption. The double blind randomised controlled trial is the most widely accepted method but in certain circumstances a less rigorous testing may be used when there are difficulties in obtaining the ideal design (Pocock, 1983).

Sceptics are always ready to recount tales of the many wonder drugs and the surgical procedures that were hailed as 'dramatic advances' and promised a new lease of life to sufferers, only to have passed into history. Many current forms of treatment were introduced years ago and although widespread in their acceptance, lack proof of their effectiveness. However, it is now very difficult to introduce a large scale clinical trial. It is to prevent such repetition of uncertainty that much greater pressure exists to 'prove' the value of any new product before it is granted the necessary approval and licensing. Thus pharmaceutical companies are extremely anxious to show not only that their products are effective in treating this particular condition, but also that they contribute to the general good of the community, as was shown by the title of a conference held in 1983 Measuring the Social Benefits of Medicine (Teeling Smith, 1983).

Heart transplantation provides an excellent example of the introduction of a new intervention procedure. It is used in the treatment of a serious stage of a common degenerative disease for which there is no proven effective treatment. Heart transplantation is a major surgical operation requiring a specialised team and extensive back-up facilities. There is considerable expense associated with the operation, the recovery period and the requirement for continuing chemotherapy. At present the operation is carried out in only a few specialised centres in the United Kingdom and there has been limited evidence of its value in terms of quantity and quality of life in the highly selected patients who have received heart transplants. Thus it would appear mandatory that a thorough evaluation be carried out before expansion of the existing limited programme could be recommended, or indeed before a decision is made to withdraw development funds. Since government funding was involved in the pilot programme, a formal study was requested by the Department of Health to identify and carry out a detailed analysis of the resource requirements and thus the costs of the current heart transplant programmes at Papworth and Harefield hospitals and to relate these to appropriate indicators of patient benefits (Buxton, Acheson, Caine, Gibson and O'Brien, 1985).

This remit illustrates the comprehensive approach to evaluation that is required of new procedures with the emphasis on costs and benefits. In this case a full epidemiological study of present and likely future demand for the procedure was not included and the ideal research design was not possible. A randomised controlled study was not established, indeed a proper non-randomised control group did not exist. The research team was able only to include in the study those who had been assessed for transplant and full analysis was limited to those accepted for transplantation. The choice of outcome measure may be a dilemma in any study since it is unlikely that any single measure will be sufficient. Survival is obviously the first outcome measure in life-threatening conditions while in certain medical problems, the expected outcome may be the reduction of a single sign or symptom such as breathlessness, tremor or skin irritation. For more serious conditions, with potentially more powerful therapy, especially where the treatment may produce certain side effects, the incorporation into the battery of outcome measures of a general instrument for the assessment of health status, which has been tested in other populations, may be a useful addition to very specific and perhaps specially designed measures. These specific measures may include such assessments as joint mobility, walking distance, impact on family relationships or degree of pain, as well as various clinical assessments. The Nottingham Health Profile was selected by the research team in the heart transplant study as a general measure of outcome because it fulfilled the criteria that had been considered appropriate for the task: that is

1. Any measure had to be sensitive to a wide range of health states, and appropriate to patients both before and after transplant.
2. The process of assessment had to be acceptable to patients, and any questions easily and unambiguously understood.
3. Preferably, it would be possible to elicit the necessary information by post, rather than merely by direct interview.
4. For purposes of comparison, the measure should have been used, or should be likely to be used, in studies of other relevant groups.
5. The choice had to ensure that a minimum of development work would be required so that the assessment of patients could be commenced as quickly as possible, and the

> system of collection and analysis of the
> data had to be consistent with available
> resources.

The research team had been:

> Struck by the grave imbalance between the
> massive literature stressing the importance of
> using health status measures in evaluative
> research, and the handful of even partially
> acceptable instruments that had actually been
> developed for such measurement to the point
> where they could be applied.

(Buxton et al, 1985)

The NHP was used to provide the following measures:

1. Perceived health status before and after
   transplantation.
2. Comparison of treated patient with
   population norms.
3. Assessment over a longer period of time
   after transplantation.

The NHP was administered to patients as part of
a longer interview at their initial assessment for
transplantation and again at any further assessments
or at pre-operative admissions. Patients awaiting
transplants were sent the questionnaire by mail at
three monthly intervals. After transplantation,
NHP's were again completed at three monthly
intervals.

The overall effect of transplantation may be
seen in Figures 7.4 to 7.9 constructed from the
summary data on Part I of the NHP. Each histogram
represents the mean scores obtained from all
observations at each point of measurement before and
after transplantation. As the authors of the report
point out it appears to suggest a single major shift
to lower scores representing an improvement in
health following transplantation. Analysis of these
scores as shown in Table 7.5 shows that in all six
sections of Part I of the NHP, the subjective health
status of individuals showed significant improvement
($P < 0.01$) with the greatest improvement in the
domain of physical mobility. Similar improvement
was noted in Part II (Table 7.6) where it is seen
that the proportion affirming that health was
affecting aspects of their life fell significantly
($P < 0.05$). The greatest reduction was in jobs

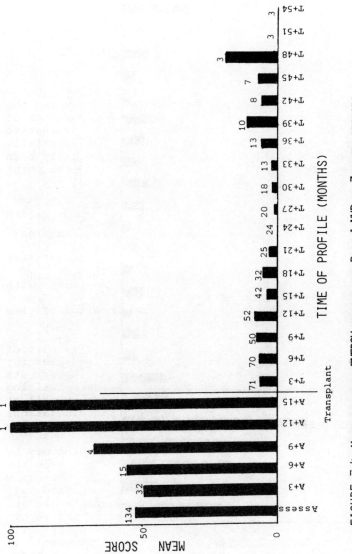

FIGURE 7.4: MEAN SCORE ON ENERGY SECTION OF PART I NHP BY 3 MONTH PERIODS
FROM INITIAL ASSESSMENT AND FROM TRANSPLANT
(number of observations above bars)

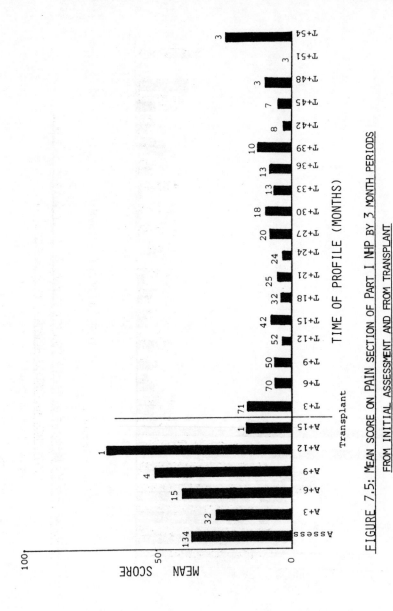

FIGURE 7.5: MEAN SCORE ON PAIN SECTION OF PART I NHP BY 3 MONTH PERIODS
FROM INITIAL ASSESSMENT AND FROM TRANSPLANT

(number of observations above bars)

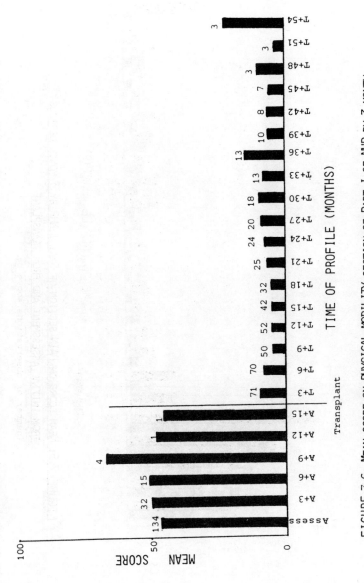

FIGURE 7.6: MEAN SCORE ON PHYSICAL MOBILITY SECTION OF PART I OF NHP BY 3 MONTH
PERIODS FROM INITIAL ASSESSMENT AND FROM TRANSPLANT

(number of observations above bars)

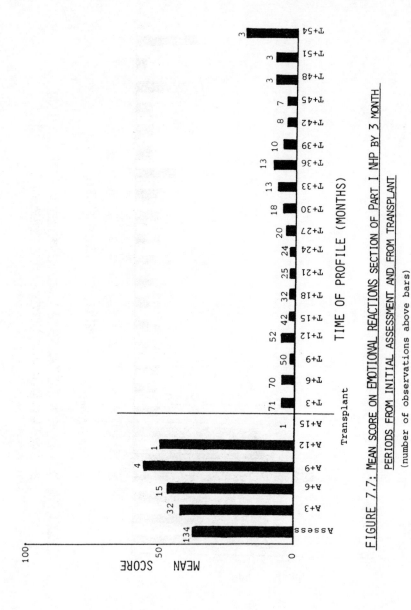

FIGURE 7.7: MEAN SCORE ON EMOTIONAL REACTIONS SECTION OF PART I NHP BY 3 MONTH PERIODS FROM INITIAL ASSESSMENT AND FROM TRANSPLANT

(number of observations above bars)

188

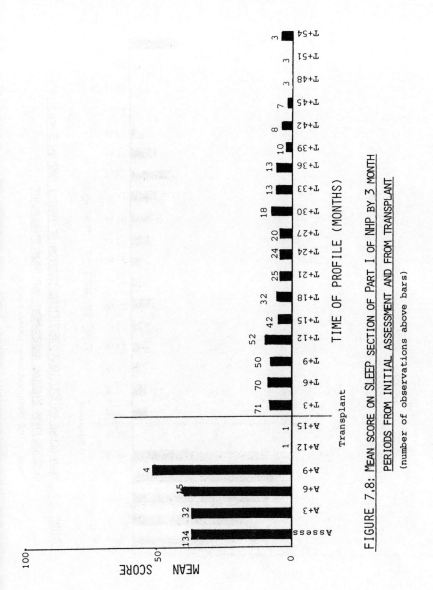

FIGURE 7.8: MEAN SCORE ON SLEEP SECTION OF PART I OF NHP BY 3 MONTH
PERIODS FROM INITIAL ASSESSMENT AND FROM TRANSPLANT

(number of observations above bars)

189

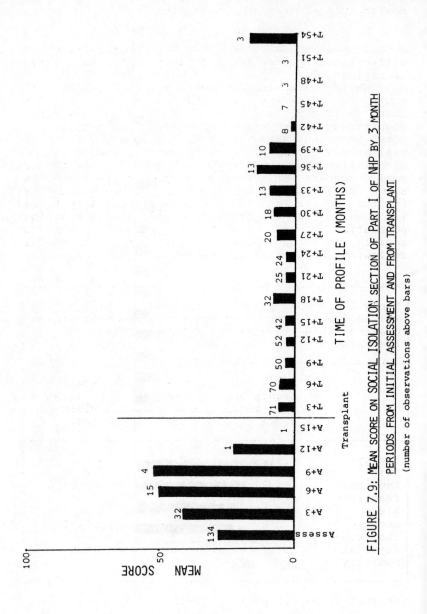

FIGURE 7.9: MEAN SCORE ON SOCIAL ISOLATION: SECTION OF PART I OF NHP BY 3 MONTH
PERIODS FROM INITIAL ASSESSMENT AND FROM TRANSPLANT

(number of observations above bars)

around the house where 82 per cent experienced difficulties prior to and only 10 per cent after transplant.

While such improvements appear dramatic, it would be surprising considering the severity of cases accepted for transplant if there was not a significant improvement in those who survive. A more important question is how does the state of health achieved relate to the normal health of men of similar age? Although there are problems of small numbers in certain age groups, it seems, as shown in Table 7.7, that there is a broad similarity in the scores of the 45-49 age group (where there is a sizeable sample) as compared with a normal population except for physical mobility, pain and social isolation where patients at three months following transplant appear to have more problems.

Table 7.5: Nottingham Health Profile, Part I: Paired Comparisons of affirmative Responses to Questions Pre-transplant and Three Months Post-transplant. Combined Hospital Data (n=62)

	Pre-transplant mean rank score	Post-transplant mean rank score	2-Tailed P value (Wilcoxon test)
Energy	27.21	18.00	< 0.01
Pain	24.65	12.25	< 0.01
Emotional reactions	31.22	12.25	< 0.01
Sleep	30.71	11.05	< 0.01
Social isolation	23.86	3.88	< 0.01
Physical mobility	32.29	5.50	< 0.01

(Adapted from Buxton et al, 1985)

The next question that must be asked is how does health status change over longer time periods following transplant? Is the initial improvement maintained and are there further improvements? The data suggests that there is no evidence of change over time. There is an indication of slow

Table 7.6: Nottingham Health Profile, Part II: Paired Comparisons of Affirmative Responses to Questions Pre-transplant and Three Months Post-transplant. Combined Hospital Data (n=62).

	Pre-transplant %	3 months post transplant %	2-tailed P value (McNemar test)
Area of life:			
Occupation	53	18	< 0.01
Jobs around the home	82	10	< 0.01
Social life	87	13	< 0.01
Home life	60	2	< 0.01
Sex life	71	24	< 0.01
Hobbies	81	19	< 0.01
Holidays	85	23	< 0.01

(Adapted from Buxton et al, 1985).

improvement in scores, but also of some higher scores on certain sections of the NHP although none of these are statistically significant. Thus in summary, the NHP indicates a clear improvement in perceived health status following the operation, leading to a near normal pattern of perceived health in relation to age. This improvement continued for the twelve month period of the study.

It should be borne in mind, however, that the sample of men studied represents only those patients who were referred to one of the two treatment centres under study; who fulfilled the selection criteria to go forward for assessment; who were selected as being suitable for transplant; who survived the period of waiting prior to transplant and who finally went for the operation.

The choice of recipients for cardiac trans-plantation is, naturally, restricted to those who are strong enough to survive until the time when a suitable donor heart becomes available. Conversely, there is some bias in the opposite direction in so far as positive clinical decisions to operate tend to favour the sickest of the remaining eligible patients. Nevertheless, it is clear that this is a highly selected group of patients and it may well be

Table 7.7: Nottingham Health Profile. Part I. Three Month Post-transplant Mean Scores (C) by Age Group (Males only) as compared with a Normal Population (P).

Age groups:		Energy	Pain	Emotional reaction	Sleep	Social isolation	Physical mobility
20-24 (n=1)	(C)	0	20.9	0	0	20.1	12.6
	(P)	10.1	0.7	11.6	8.4	5.5	1.5
25-29 (n=3)	(C)	0	0	5.6	0	0	0
	(P)	8.6	1.6	10.3	8.6	5.6	1.6
30-34 (n=4)	(C)	6.0	0	2.4	6.3	0	0
	(P)	4.0	2.8	6.3	6.2	2.9	1.3
35-39 (n=4)	(C)	6.0	4.3	0	3.1	0	0
	(P)	5.0	2.6	10.3	5.7	2.7	1.2
40-44 (n=17)	(C)	4.5	9.8	7.7	5.0	9.4	16.5
	(P)	10.1	5.8	10.4	11.9	5.0	3.2
45-49 (n=22)	(C)	8.8	6.0	6.0	8.4	6.4	13.3
	(P)	8.0	3.0	7.7	8.4	1.6	1.1
50-54 (n=11)	(C)	6.5	4.5	6.2	25.8	2.0	6.8
	(P)	11.6	7.1	10.6	13.4	5.5	4.1
55-59 (n=3)	(C)	8.0	0	0	4.2	0	3.7
	(P)	13.3	2.9	7.7	11.7	3.4	3.7

(Adapted from Buxton et al, 1985)

that quality of life after transplantation is much better in this group than it would be if, say, all those who needed new hearts could get them immediately and survive. Patients who are recommended for cardiac transplantation have to be thought suitable in the first place in terms of the probability of them standing up to the operation itself. If one adds to this their capacity to survive the waiting period it is possible that the patients described here are a particularly robust sub-sample of the total number of men with severe cardiovascular disease, certainly they represent a restricted age range; only three patients were aged over 55 years.

Notwithstanding these remarks, the addition of reliable and valid quality of life measures to outcome and process evaluation can bring an important new perspective to the understanding of the effects of radical medical intervention. In general, it can be said that instruments such as the Nottingham Health Profile constitute valuable adjuncts to clinical assessments. From the point of view of medical care they serve to direct attention to aspects of a patient's life which might otherwise go unremarked. In so doing they open up the opportunity for timely counselling or other support services and can highlight undesirable and unsuspected side effects. In addition such measures provide standard scores by means of which valid comparisons can be made both within and between groups.

Further analyses from this study are proceeding and will examine the relationship between scores on the NHP at initial assessment interviews and other outcome measures, for example, mortality after acceptance but prior to transplantation; adjustment to post-transplant living. Differences in initial scores between those men who were rejected and those who were definitely or provisionally accepted, prognosis and outcome will be computed and individual differences in perceived health will be scrutinised in order to see if it is possible to identify factors important in coping.

Clearly, it would be of great interest to have a reliable means of predicting suitability for cardiac transplantation, probability of survival and transplantation sequelae based upon patients' perceptions, which would supplement clinical judgements.

In studies of surgical procedures or the effects of chemotherapy, not only is there the

possibility of examining improvement or
deterioration in perceived health following a
particular procedure, but, in randomised controlled
trials, this could be compared either with no
treatment or with some existing treatment. This
might show different rates of recovery or different
outcomes in selected domains. The NHP is more
sensitive and standardised than the traditional
measures of recovery, such as time of return to work
or resumption of normal social activities (Finlayson
and McEwen, 1971). The NHP could also assist in
detecting the recurrence of problems and, perhaps,
indicate the beginning of a relapse so that
intervention could be swiftly applied.

MONITORING PROGRESS IN PROBLEMATIC SITUATIONS

A further possible application of the Profile is to
groups of patients where there is considerable
uncertainty of prognosis. Cancer patients are an
example of such a group. Individuals or certain
categories of patients may be at higher risk of
psychological disturbance in the early stages of
clinical treatment and therefore, might benefit from
specialised care and support. In addition, in the
longer term, the NHP might assist in monitoring
progress and adding an additional perspective to
clinical assessments, which might help inform the
direction of further therapy. The special problems
of toxicity and side effects associated with
cytotoxic therapy were noted by Priestman (1984)
especially where this is used following surgical
treatment to treat possible micrometastasis. He
described two measures which give accurate and
sensitive assessments of measuring subjective
toxicity but considered that, although these may
give an indication of quality of life, further
refinement was needed. A preliminary study of the
use of the NHP with cancer patients illustrates this
approach (Moriarty and Hunt, 1984). The sample
consisted of patients attending a clinic in a Dublin
hospital.

Of 63 new patients attending for radiotherapy
it was found that approximately 20 per cent
experienced little or no evidence of distress as
measured by the NHP. The remaining 80 per cent had
poor subjective health status with some of the
highest levels of distress possible, especially in
emotional reactions, lack of energy and sleep.
There appeared to be a relationship between

perceived health at diagnosis and at the end of therapy with those with the worst problems at diagnosis showing little improvement after treatment.

Patients with skin cancer showed least distress in perceived health at time of diagnosis and there was a considerable improvement following treatment. The data suggested that diagnosis engenders a great deal of emotional distress, particularly in females, but much of this has dissipated by the start of treatment. In a group of patients with residual or recurrent disease (19 patients) there were lower levels of perceived discomfort and distress than with new patients, but poor perceived health in the domains of sleep and energy for men and emotional reactions and social isolation for women. There also appeared to be more disability in daily life although this may reflect the fact that they formed an older age group.

In a small group of patients (14) who were attending follow-up and who had no residual disease the scores were fairly low. In all categories of cancer patients there was considerable range in scores on the NHP, with some individuals having high or very high scores. A comparison of patients with cancers at different sites is shown in Figure 7.10. Such analyses may allow individuals with special needs to be detected and within each disease grouping extra support can be given to those with the greatest expressed problems. This may allow extra help to be given to those who do not complain as well as those who are more vocal in expressing their problems. Molleman and his colleagues (1984) have indicated the importance of expert help in providing information and in assisting the patient and his or her close relative in reducing anxiety.

THE POTENTIAL VALUE OF THE NOTTINGHAM HEALTH PROFILE

Although these are preliminary studies and further work is required to confirm the impressions gained, it would appear that the NHP has a value in helping to decide on the 'best' treatment, identifying categories of patients, or types of therapy where outcome is less satisfactory, identifying groups of patients at particular risk and assisting with the monitoring of progress. It would appear that in clinical situations there is a potential benefit to providers of care, patients and planners.

As with all tools there are limitations and

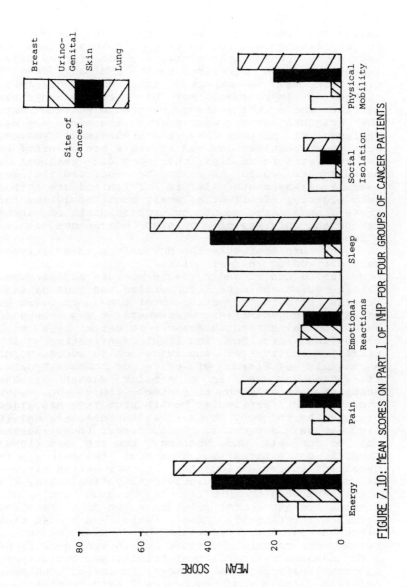

FIGURE 7.10: MEAN SCORES ON PART I OF NHP FOR FOUR GROUPS OF CANCER PATIENTS

197

there are likely to be situations where the NHP may be of little or no benefit. It is a relatively severe measure and, therefore, may not pick up minor improvements in perceived health and many forms of treatment may be expected to produce only small changes. Improvement may be perceived by the patient where there is no change in score because the original score was zero. The NHP was not designed to pick up changes in individual symptoms such as breathlessness and if these are required to be evaluated in studies, then specific questions or measurements would have to be included in any overall assessment. It is of limited use in the very elderly, frail or severely handicapped and for these groups assessment by professionals or carers may be the only way of obtaining indications of change.

For professionals the NHP offers an additional perspective to normal clinical assessments. It provides a valid and reliable measure of perceived health which could be incorporated into the patient records allowing comparison over time. It could be of value in general practice where it might be used as an initial screening measure to detect those with ill-defined problems who might benefit from health promotion activities involving health education or a variety of forms of medical or community care. It could be used in a similar manner in the occupational setting to detect those who might profit from a particular health promotion programme designed by the occupational health team. It can be used to assess progress and to detect those who are not doing well and who may require additional support or alternative treatment following more detailed investigation of the poor health status. As well as its use in individual patient care, the Nottingham Health Profile can be used in clinical studies to assess the relative value of alternative forms of treatment. Greer (1984) has argued that since a cardinal principle of medical ethics is primum non nocere, failure to include quality of life assessments in clinical trials, particularly in cancer treatment, is a major omission and that detailed measures of psychosocial adjustment should be included in all future trials of cancer therapy. Although it has never been used in a double blind randomised controlled trial, the NHP would seem to be a suitable tool for inclusion in such a study. There would be no special requirements other than those normally attached to such trials and indeed, the ethical imperative to carry out such studies before the introduction of a new therapeutic regimen would indicate a requirement to obtain a measure of health status by some appropriate means. The NHP would appear to have a potential in predicting outcome of care. If the features of those who do badly on a particular form of intervention can be identified then these individuals could be investigated and alternative forms of treatment offered. The importance of the doctor-patient relationship in chronic disease is well-recognised (Ben-Sira, 1984) and the provision of additional information to the doctor on the patient's perspective could do much to improve the quality of their relationship and hence lead to improved care and improved response.

There is considerable debate on the benefits and risks of giving patients access to their own clinical records, either to look at or to keep (Shenkin and Warner, 1973, Metcalfe, 1980). Those in favour of this feel that the benefits of greater knowledge, the sense of participation and partnership that the patient would experience, would lead to more effective health care. A health profile would seem to provide a way of achieving this. If patients had a simple visual record of their profile, which might be administered to them on appropriate occasions and the relationship between this and treatment decision explained, then the concept of effective partnership between patient and professional in health care might be more easily achieved. It could also be of value to those committed to self-help and who need to strengthen their arguments for improvements in health service provision (Hatch and Kickbusch, 1983).

For those involved in the planning and provision of health care, the determination of priorities and decisions on the introduction of new forms of care, the NHP would provide a standard method that could be incorporated into wider epidemiological assessments and the estimation of costs and benefits. Williams (1984) argues that the doctor as clinician, practice manager and general policy maker must have a more comprehensive view of what is ethical, moving away from the gross inadequacy of the common view that the prime ethical imperative in medicine is to do all that is possible for the patient who consults him, to an ethic based on cost-benefit principles.

Most of the studies reported here indicate the potential of the Nottingham Health Profile, but this could be realised only if there is strict adherence to research design in future planned studies. The haphazard administration of questionnaires to unselected patients may be easy but will be of no value. The study design must take account of the very ill patient, the elderly confused person, the young child or the immigrant who may not be capable of completing it, or understanding it and for whom it may not have been tested or validated. The tempting simplicity of using the NHP should not mean that it is used without thought.

Not only is there need to evaluate new forms of treatment, but there are many conditions which have either a long established but uncertain remedy or where there is a plethora of treatments which indicate a lack of proof. In many instances choice is based on clinical judgement and it will be interesting to see if, when 'subjective' data on perceived health is produced from well designed clinical studies, this alters prescribing patterns.

REFERENCES

Ben-Sira, Z. (1984) 'Chronic Illness, Stress and Coping', Soc Sci Med, 18, 725-736

Buxton, M. Acheson, R. Caine, R. Gibson, S. and O'Brien, B. (1985) Costs and Benefits of the Heart Transplant Programmes at Harefield and Papworth Hospitals, Research Report No. 12, DHSS, HMSO, London

Cay, E.L. Philip, A.E. Small, W.P. Neilson, J. and and Henderson, M.A. (1975) 'Patients' Assessment of the Result of Surgery for Peptic Ulcer', Lancet, 1, 29-31

Conrad, P. (1985) 'The Meaning of Medications: Another Look at Compliance', Soc Sci Med, 20, 29-37

Dunnell, K. and Cartwright, A. (1972) Medicine Takers, Prescribers and Hoarders, Routledge and Kegan Paul, London

Finlayson, A. and McEwen, J. (1977) Coronary Heart Disease and Patterns of Living, Croom Helm, London

Greer, S. (1984) 'The Psychological Dimension in Cancer Treatment', Soc Sci Med, 18, 345-349

Hall, R. Horrocks, J.C. Clamp, S.E. and Dombal, D.T. (1976) 'Observer Variation in Assessment of Results of Surgery for Peptic Ulceration', BMJ 1, 814-816

Hatch, S. and Kickbusch, I. (1983) Self-help and Health in Europe, WHO, Copenhagen

Himsworth, R.L. (1985) 'The Appropriate Use of Diagnostic Services, (iii) Thyroid Disease and the Laboratory Health Trends', 17, 25-26

Hunt, S.M. McEwen, J. McKenna S.P. Backett, E.M. and Pope, C. (1984) 'Subjective Health Assessments and the Perceived Outcome of Minor Surgery', J Psychosom Res, 28, 105-114

Kitzinger, S. (1972) The Experience of Childbirth, Penguin, Harmondsworth

Leifer, M. (1977) Psychological Changes accompanying Pregnancy and Motherhood, Genetic Monographs, 95

Lubin, B. Gardener, S.H. and Roth, A. (1975) 'Mood and Somatic Symptoms during Pregnancy', Psychosom Med, 37, 138-145

Lumley, J. (1978) 'Sexual Feelings in Pregnancy and after Childbirth', Aust NZ J Obstet Gynaecol, 18, 114

McColl, I. Drinkwater, J.E. Hulme-Moir, I. and Donnan, S.P.B. (1971) 'Prediction of Success and Failure in Gastric Surgery', Brit J Surg, 58, 768-771

Macy, C. and Faulkner, F. (1979) Pregnancy and Birth. Pleasures and Problems, Harper and Row, Row, London

Metcalfe, D.H.H. (1980) ' Why not let the Patients keep their own Records?', J Roy Coll Gen Pract, 30, 420

Molleman, E. Krabbendam, P.J. Annyas, A.A. Koops, H.S. Sleijer, D.T. and Vermey, A. (1984) 'The Signficance of the Doctor-Patient Relationship in Coping with Cancer', Soc Sci Med, 18, 475-480

Moriarty, M. and Hunt, S.M. (1984) 'Use of a Measure of Perceived Health with Cancer Patients', Unpublished report

Pockcok, S.J. (1983) Clinical Trials: A Practical Approach, John Wiley Chichester

Priestman, T.J. (1984) 'Quality of Life after Cytotoxic Chemotherapy: Discussion Paper', J Roy Soc Med, 77, 492-495

Sackett, D.L. Haynes, R.B. and Tugwell, P. (1985) Clinical Epidemiology: A Basic Source for Clinical Medicine, Little, Brown and Co, Boston

Schacht, P.J. and Pemberton, A. (1985) 'What is Unnecessary Surgery? Who shall decide? Issue of Consumer Sovereignty, Conflict and Self-Regulation', Soc Sci Med, 21, 199-206

Shenkin, B.N. and Warner, D.C. (1973) 'Giving the Patient his Medical Record. A Proposal to improve the System', <u>New Eng J Med</u>, <u>89</u>, 688-692

Teeling Smith, G. (1983) <u>Measuring the Social Benefits of Medicine</u>, Office of Health Economics, London

Williams, A. (1984) Medical Ethics, Health Service Efficiency and Clinical Freedom, <u>Nuffield/York Portfolio No. 2</u>, Nuffield Provincial Hospitals Trust, London

Williams, J. Lindsay, J, Hunt, S.M. and McKenna, S.P. (1981) 'Perceived Health during Pregnancy', Unpublished data

Chapter 8.

CROSS-CULTURAL ISSUES IN HEALTH INDICATORS

So far, the main emphasis in this book has been upon the use of health status measurement in Britain and the United States. However, since all member countries of the World Health Organisation have agreed to encourage the development and use of indicators of health, disease and disability as a basis for the planning of services, it is important that the discussion be widened to encompass other cultures.

The vast majority of health indicators, whether compiled from routine statistics or developed from survey research have had their inception in Western Europe and the United States. The use of these indicators in other countries and cultures may be seen as desirable for two reasons:

1. To enable other countries to gather information on the health status of their own population.
2. To make cross-cultural comparisons.

It is clear that if cross-cultural comparisons are to be made then the health indicators in question must be equally applicable, reliable, valid and acceptable in each culture. If, however, the assessment of health status and health needs is to remain confined to a single culture or country, then the development and testing of the relevant culture-specific indicators would be more efficacious.

There is, ostensibly, no real reason why cross-cultural comparisons need to be made. Often they result in 'league-tables' of, for example, infant mortality, which serve only to underline the superior resources of the western world and give occasion for self-congratulation. The policies of the World Health Organisation have, however, led to a climate in which the use of standard indicators in all member countries is seen as desirable in terms of international policy and planning.

There are also other reasons why existing indicators might be used in cultures for which they were not developed. Firstly, the efficacy of mortality and morbidity statistics for health planning in western countries is assumed to hold for all cultures. Secondly, the development, testing and standardisation of special indicators is costly and time-consuming; adaptation of an extant instrument may, therefore, be cheaper than the initiation of a new one. Thirdly, many indicators may appear, at least superficially, to have universal applicability. Attempts to adapt health indicators in one culture for use in another culture, however, are fraught with problems. These problems may be categorised as technical, conceptual and linguistic.

The generation of any sorts of data may be regarded as a social process which has its origins in the orientations, concerns and beliefs of a particular culture. The mere fact that a society comes to believe in and depend upon routinely gathered information for policy and planning implies a particular kind of 'rational' approach. Whether this approach is appropriate or even desirable in all cultures depends upon the common understanding and acceptance of the underlying <u>Weltanschauung</u>. At the present time this cannot be said to be the case.

MORTALITY RATES

Until very recently death was thought to be a rather easily ascertained and objective 'fact', thus making mortality statistics particularly attractive as indicators of a nation's health. As has been noted in chapter 3, some mortality statistics in the West are now being questioned for their reliability and use as a consequence of changing patterns of disease, increased longevity and the very low rates in some categories. Cross-cultural comparisons of mortality rates must take into account variations in reliability, validity and appropriateness between countries.

Even in Europe and the United States where record keeping is embedded in a highly organised bureaucracy, it is estimated that, for example, perinatal mortality figures are either incomplete or of uncertain reliability. On the other hand, the statistics for infant mortality are regarded as acceptable for all the larger European states including the Soviet Union (United Nations, 1972).

The technical problems that account for variations in reliability stem from uncertainties about definitions, for example, perinatal death is that which occurs between 28 weeks of gestation and one week of age - a definition on which there is not yet universal agreement, in addition to the problems of ascertainment of age.

Whereas proof of the death of an infant or an adult may be necessary, not only for legal purposes, but also to obtain a burial permit, ensure inheritance, family allowances, or insurance, such that importance is given to the time, place and manner of death, the loss of a foetus may be regarded as of lesser importance. In addition, where there is no central registration system, procedures for collating death statistics become problematic. Reliable perinatal rates can only be assumed under conditions where early and regular ante-natal care is available from official agencies and, preferably, where the majority of births take place in hospital. However, even under these conditions, there is much room for error, in particular, in the distinction between stillbirth, abortion and livebirth.

The technical issues associated with the reliable collection of mortality statistics loom large in non-industrialised countries. In areas of the world where the continuing existence of parasitic and infectious diseases, as well as malnutrition, accounts for the major number of deaths, mortality figures are particularly useful indicators of the nation's health - or rather lack of it. However, such areas are also likely to lack the resources to keep such figures accurately. People in remote rural areas, or overcrowded urban areas may fail to report the death of a child, or even an adult. Administrative centres where figures can be stored may not exist or be inefficient. Cultural practices and traditional beliefs may sanction alternative means of dealing with death than those officially recommended. Lack of trained personnel may make cause of death hard to ascertain and medical diagnosis may be less of a priority to parents than the socio-cultural meaning of the loss. In fact, cause-of-death statistics are, at present, either very deficient or non-existent for most of the world's population. Hospital statistics, in addition to the usual drawbacks, are usually very inadequate in non-industrialised countries, if they are kept at all. Where resources are scarce, the provision of trained clerical personnel will not receive high priority. The very young and the very old are the least likely to be medically attended in hospitals, so that data for the extremes of the age range are likely to be unavailable.

It should also be borne in mind that a concern with some indicators, such as perinatal mortality say, reflects the significance of such an event in affluent countries. Premature loss of a child may be of much less importance where the birth and death rates are high. An overall child mortality rate, as suggested by Murnaghan (1981) might be more useful in such cases. Even so, the task of keeping track of infant and adult deaths may be herculean in non-industrialised countries and has led to a search for alternatives. For example, Blom (1981), in West Zambia, attempted to construct a 'survival index' based upon the assumption that a mother would surely know how many children she had given birth to and how many had survived. Thus, for groups of women with the same gravidity the mean number of children still alive could be calculated and used as a crude index of need for perinatal and infant health services. A major drawback of such a system is, of course, the relatively large numbers of mothers who also die and are thus unavailable to report. A study in Nigeria demonstrated the efficacy and lower cost of household surveys for collecting vital statistics as an alternative to central registration and recording (Aleyni and Oloyinka, 1978).

MORBIDITY

Ascertainment of the incidence and prevalence of morbidity in many countries poses even more problems. It is notoriously difficult even where a centrally organised body exists for collecting the data. In some areas individuals suffer multiple conditions, but only one may be apparent. Some states may be regarded as socially undesirable by both lay people and medical personnel, for example, suicide abortion, venereal disease, and will tend to be under-reported. Diagnoses depend upon social processes relating to labelling and the manner of presentation of symptoms. The reporting of some conditions may be discouraged or distorted for political or economic reasons. For example, an outbreak of cholera might seriously affect tourism and a great deal of minor and even major illness is more likely to go unremarked where there are no facilities for treating it.

The cross-cultural uses of indicators such as restricted activity, incapacity, or sickness absence make little sense in societies where such events are a consequence of variations in illness perception, role requirements and employment patterns.

SOCIO-MEDICAL INDICATORS

In addition to the technical and conceptual problems so evident in the case of mortality and morbidity statistics, socio-medical indicators add the further issue of linguistics, as well as highlighting further dimensions of the conceptual problems.

As was pointed out in chapter 4, even within the same culture there is much ambiguity and lack of consensus, concerning the presence or absence of 'health', 'illness' and 'disease'. Cross-culturally this ambiguity is compounded by differences in the meaning systems of cultures and their historical development. Socialisation into a culture involves the internationalisation of the prevailing social reality - a reality which is constructed by that society in so far as certain interpretations, events, meanings, patterns and behaviours are regarded as legitimate, whilst others are not (Berger and Luckman, 1965). In very small societies social reality is likely to be shared by all the members. In larger heterogeneous and pluralistic societies, varying realities may co-exist, but with each group having some knowledge of the others. Naturally, meanings attached to health and illness are embedded in the matrix of social reality. The experience of illness is a cultural phenomenon which is reflected in beliefs about aetiology, manifest- ation of symptoms and illness behaviour, roles assigned to the relevant players, goals and methods of treatment and the evaluation of outcome.

Thus signs, symptoms, statements and behaviour indicative of health problems will be intimately related to the meanings assigned to health within that culture or subculture and the prevailing concepts concerning aetiology.

For instance, among the Sepik in New Guinea, illness is defined according to the presumed causal agent which may be mystical or human. Consequently, the presence of illness depends much more upon the social and moral status of the patient and his or her relationships than it does upon symptoms (Lewis, 1975). Similarly, among the Safwa of Tanzania, illness is believed to be a consequence of a weakening of the life force caused by social disharmony. Indicators of disease may thus be sought in family or kinship discord. Diagnostic techniques are focused on the community rather than on the individual and are directed to ascertaining the reason for the disharmony rather than the name of the malady. Not infrequently, remedies will be applied after the death of the patient, whose fate is less important than the re-establishment of harmonious relationships (Harwood, 1970).

In addition to internationally classified disorders and diseases, there exist culture-specific conditions and folk illnesses, for example 'Susto' in Mexico and some parts of Latin America, a disorder characterised by anorexia, insomnia and trembling believed to be caused by the entry of magical substances into the body and leading to 'soul loss'. 'Kayakangst' is confined to the Eskimos of West Greenland and 'Witiko' to the Indians of NE Canada. Such conditions have implications and expectations attached to them which are unique to the culture, as are the actions taken in their treatment. Moral, ethical and social indicators are likely to be more relevant than medical ones.

Different cultural values and experiences also mean that conditions regarded as evidence of disease in one culture may not be so regarded in others. In certain parts of Africa intestinal worms are so common as to seem normal. Some middle-eastern cultures look on obesity as a sign of good health, affluence and beauty. Within British society occurences regarded as normal by one section of the population would be abhorred by another. For example, morning cough may be thought quite desirable in parts of the north of England since it is believed to 'clear the tubes'. Chronic fatigue may become so familiar as to go unremarked and feeling tired would not be regarded as symptomatically significant.

Another aspect of conceptual differences is the way in which malaise may be expressed. For example some Chinese groups have learned to place a taboo on the public expression of emotion especially where it is strong and negative in nature. Such emotions are regarded as destructive to the harmonious family relationships which are the bedrock and preoccupation of traditional Chinese life (Hsu, 1971).

Family and ancestor worship are an integral part of the culture, the family is believed to exist prior to and after the death of any individual member and must be kept inviolate since it ensures continuity of past, present and future. This is reflected in the language itself. Hokkien and Chinese, although well endowed with terms for bodily states, are relatively impoverished in relation to psychological terminology. Kleiman, Eisenberg and Good (1978) in their studies of the Taiwanese, have pointed out how the expression of ideas and feelings are divided into public and private; the former being somewhat shallow and unrevealing, whilst the latter are implicitly personal and unlikely to be revealed, for example, to a doctor, sociologist or health researcher. The obverse of this occurs amongst the Subanun of the Philippines who love to talk about how they feel and are very knowledgeable about disease. Unfortunately (for indicator reliability and validity) they rarely depend upon their own perceptions, but actively seek the opinion of family, friends, neighbours and others before deciding upon their health status - thus diagnosis is essentially communal (Frake, 1961).

A reluctance or inability to express socio-emotional distress appears to be quite common and in many non-industrialised societies, emotional problems tend to be somatised and expressed in terms of physiological malfunctioning (Leff, 1977). This has also been observed among working class people in Europe, especially men. Thus emotional problems may be presented as headache, diarrhoea, tachycardia, backpain or tremor, for example. There appear to be two main reasons for this: firstly, the non-salience of psychological problems in societies where life is physically very hard and merely subsisting leaves little time for pondering one's inner mental states; and secondly, where the culture abhors expressions of anxiety, depression and anger as socially disruptive such that anyone who expresses such negative emotions is threatened with social dishonour and isolation. In addition, men may be more likely to somatise complaints where emotional expression is regarded as unmanly.

In Saudi Arabia women are brought up to be passive and highly dependent and expected to create and maintain a calm atmosphere in the home. Consequently, feelings of unhappiness or dissatis-sfaction tend to be presented physiologically in terms of fatigue, headache, loss of appetite or palpitations such that the responsibility cannot be

209

seen to lie with the woman (Racy, 1980).

Another aspect of cultural variation pertains especially to disability indicators. Impairments such as loss of a limb, sensory defects or dyslexia may or may not be handicapping conditions depending upon social, occupational and environmental demands as well as the level of technology in the culture. Thus, similar scores on a disability scale would not necessarily have the same meaning in different societies, nor would they carry the same implications for service planning.

A consideration of such cultural variations must, therefore, precede any attempt to adapt already existing instruments for use in a culture or with a sub-group whose members were not included in the testing and standardisation process of the indicator. An increase in the reliability of mortality rates may require merely enhanced communication, training and the addition of extra resources; reliable and valid socio-medical instruments that can be used cross-culturally will require the closest attention to the technical, conceptual and linguistic issues implicit in differing social contingencies.

QUESTIONNAIRES AND INTERVIEWS

The use of questionnaires and interviews to obtain health status information is so fully accepted in western countries that it is easy to forget that it depends upon several pre-suppositions: that the majority of the people are literate, that the respondents share common values in relation to health and that these methods of questioning will be understandable and acceptable, both in the form of the questions and the range of possible responses. Standardised questions and forced choice answers may be quite alien to someone who is unfamiliar with them and who has not been socialised into a 'survey society'. As has been noted, many cultures encourage a reluctance to answer personal questions and there are groups where an individual will refuse to answer unless a third party is present (Mitchell, 1968). Motivation to complete a questionnaire or interview cannot be assumed. Another technical problem arises where the instrument consists of scaled items. Priorities, notions of severity and values are different in different cultures. Weights assigned in one culture are thus likely to be quite inappropriate in another.

Self report instruments will also fail where there is a low level of literacy or where, as among the Subanun, discussion with others precedes labelling of one's own conditions, physical or mental.

Conceptual and Linguistic Issues

Socio-medical indicators found to be useful in one culture and which are being considered for use in another must be submitted to rigorous examination for conceptual, semantic and linguistic equivalence.

Many cross-cultural studies have shown a careless attitude to translation. For example, the National Health Interview Survey in the USA and the General Household Survey in Britain have generally relied upon bilingual relatives and friends for instantaneous translation to non-English speaking respondents. This could have unknown and probably profound effects upon the validity and reliability of the information obtained.

Very few standardised socio-medical indicators have been conscientiously translated from one language to another, and much knowledge in this area is drawn from the field of intelligence testing, where one of three strategies for adaptation is usually adopted; the development of a set of measures supposedly applicable in all cultures; the construction of instruments usable in all cultures, but supplemented by country specific items; or the use of items which are semantically different and where interpretations are confined to the particular setting and no cross-cultural comparisons are made.

Translation

Literal translation of items into another language seeks to maintain a one-to-one correspondence whilst allowing for necessary changes in word order and syntax required by the grammar. However, this raises the issue of the 'functional equivalency' of words and concepts in the two languages. Matesanz (1974) has pointed out that a lack of congruence in the meaning of concepts and the implications of differences in meaning may necessitate the substitution of expressions which are equivalent rather than identical.

Conceptual and semantic equivalence are not necessarily the same. With equivalence of meaning, translated questions mean more or less the same thing, but conceptual equivalence implies that responses to questions are indicative of the same concept. For example, 'I have pain in my head' may be translated with semantic equivalence, but the significance of an affirmative response may be quite different in different cultures. Accordingly, a particular indicator may, when translated, show:

1. Both conceptual and semantic equivalence, in which case the translated items are identical.
2. Neither conceptual nor semantic equivalence, in which case the items are unusable.
3. Conceptual, but not semantic equivalence, in which case the mode of expression needs to be changed.
4. Semantic but not conceptual equivalence, in which case the items are culture-linked and the significance of responses needs to be reconsidered.

(Bice and Kalimo, 1971).

Some examples of semantic equivalence, but not conceptual being achieved can be seen in the use of the Cornell Medical Index (CMI) with Alaskan Eskimo and Vietnamese respondents. The Index has a section which attempts to tap feelings of inadequacy, one of the items asks, 'Do you always feel like you need someone to help you make up your mind?' Eskimo females are expected to play a passive role and consult their men folk about decisions. Thus an affirmative answer is indicative of conformity or adjustment to the culture, rather than indec- isiveness (Chance, 1962). Similarly, in a study of newly arrived Vietnamese in the USA, the CMI items which are meant to tap feelings of inadequacy in American respondents rather point up aspects of modesty and shyness which are highly regarded by the Vietnamese (Eyton and Neuwirth, 1984). Another example is drawn from the use of a Social Adaptation Questionnaire, again with Vietnamese in the USA. An affirmative answer to the statement, 'I do not find it easy to make friends with Americans' is regarded as indicative of poor adjustment. However, because of the value placed on modesty and shyness (qualities which are less evident in American citizens) and severe language barriers, the meaning of a positive response is related much more to cultural and linguistic factors than social psychological ones (Vignes and Hall, 1979).

The Sapir-Whorf hypothesis, i.e. that human beings are profoundly influenced in their cognitions and perceptions by the language they use, suggests that the separate words which make up a translated questionnaire or interview item require the closest attention if they are not to prove misleading.

Werner and Campbell (1970) have suggested instructions for writing English that can be successfully translated: using simple sentences of less than sixteen words; having items in the active, rather than the passive voice; and avoiding pronouns, metaphors, colloquialisms and the subjunctive case. However, even if these conditions can be fulfilled, functional equivalency may be absent.

AN ARABIC VERSION OF THE NOTTINGHAM HEALTH PROFILE

Many of the foregoing points can be illustrated by an early attempt at translating the Nottingham Health Profile into Arabic, for use in Egypt. In 1980, under the aegis of the World Health Organisation, a project known as the 'Health Coverage Study' was set up in Egypt, Bahrain and North Yemen aimed at providing a comprehensive description of health status, health care facilities and utilisation patterns in those countries. The Institute of National Planning in Egypt, who had responsibility for the project, learned of the Nottingham Health Profile and asked if they might use it. Some reservations were expressed by the research team about the applicability of such an instrument, not only in a very different culture, but in a setting where the health issues are of a very different nature. However, it was eventually agreed to set up a pilot study, using Part I only, since Part II was clearly inapplicable.

Firstly, the items were translated by a bi-lingual Egyptian into colloquial Arabic, as used in Cairo and the Delta area. Surprisingly close semantic equivalence was achieved, but for some items it proved impossible to convey the same meaning as did the English version. For example, 'I'm feeling on edge' could be translated only as 'I am afraid'. A complicating problem was that the items would have to be asked by an interviewer, instead of being self-administered, because of the high level of illiteracy. This raised another issue – how to cope with the quite marked differences between written and spoken Arabic. Moreover, the form, intonation and complexity of Arabic expression depends upon the individual's place in the social hierarchy, and whether he or she resides in an urban or rural area, and it also differs between Upper and Lower Egypt. After much discussion a version was chosen which was thought likely to be understandable to the majority of potential respondents.

These technical problems of translation and administration were then augmented by problems of sampling. Testing sites were chosen at two rural health centres, in Omkhfnan and Tomva, and at Om El-Masrien hospital, in Giza, to obtain urban clients. However, since rural dwellers will often travel many miles to visit a well known hospital the distinction between rural and urban samples was by no means clear cut.

Examination of these samples showed them not surprisingly, to be almost totally dissimilar to those on which the Profile had been tested in England. Egyptian clients tended to be younger, disproportionately female, poor, illiterate, malnourished and consulting mainly with infectious diseases at a late stage in the illness. English health care users are mainly older, comparatively well nourished, literate, from a wide socio-economic spectrum, often with chronic conditions for which they seek early intervention. In addition, many Egyptian women attend a health clinic for social reasons, to meet friends and to get away from unpleasant home conditions.

Testing was eventually carried out on 60 people, 64 per cent of whom were female and 74 per cent of whom were illiterate. The small size of the sample resulted from unwillingness to participate, especially on the part of the comparatively more affluent urban clients and males. The sample was, therefore, predominantly a rural and female one. Respondents were asked both to respond to the items in terms of negation or affirmation and also to say what they thought the item meant. It soon became clear that the twin aims of semantic and conceptual equivalence had not been achieved for a majority of the items, and, moreover, that many items had little saliency for the respondents. Items on the emotional reactions section soon brought to light that the concern of western individuals for their psychological states was almost completely alien to the respondents. For example, the statement 'I've forgotten what it's like to enjoy myself', although it translates well enough, does not have much existential relevance in a context where the <u>concept</u> of enjoyment is not present. Living in, or on, the edge of poverty, most of the day is taken up with work, finding food, caring for children and generally subsisting, rather than with the pursuit of pleasure. The item 'I'm feeling on edge', which as stated earlier, translated as 'I am afraid' elicited distress in many respondents because of religious precepts founded in Islam which enjoin against the outward expression of fear. The statement 'I feel that life is not worth living' was regarded as sacrilegious, since life is regarded as having been given by God and individuals have no right to make such judgements. Semantic equivalence in Arabic could not be attained for 'Things are getting me down'. The translation was primarily interpreted in physical, rather than emotional terms, in the sense of being pressed into the ground or being tired at the end of the day. Only two items from the emotional section emerged relatively unscathed: 'I wake up feeling depressed' and 'I lose my temper easily these days'.

The energy section contains three statements which are easily distinguishable in meaning by English respondents. These distinctions proved hard to express in Arabic and the Egyptian respondents interpreted them as having the same meaning. The section on social isolation was found to have no relevance to respondents. Statements like 'I feel I am a burden to people' or 'I'm finding it hard to get on with people' express experiences which are absent from a daily life which is communal and mutually supportive. These kinds of statements elicited only puzzlement and occasionally horror that such situations could be imagined.

The five items on sleep were mostly understandable, but inapplicable, since scarcely anyone had problems sleeping, being rather exhausted after a long day of physical labour. A few of the eight items on physical mobility were understood and answered in the sense intended. However, other statements posed conceptual or superstitious problems. For example, 'I find it hard to dress myself' offended notions of personal privacy and apparently terrified some respondents who made comments such as 'God take such evil away from me'. A statement like 'I find it hard to stand for long' was irrelevant since most tasks are carried out sitting on the ground and very little actual standing is done.

The majority of statements on pain were easily understood, but an item involving pain on using stairs or steps was not appropriate since such obstacles are rarely encountered in a rural setting.

This example demonstrates very well the pitfalls of such an exercise in attempting to adapt a socio-medical indicator devloped in one culture for use in another, very different culture. The conceptual world of an Egyptian peasant scarcely encompasses the daily health concerns of an English citizen or vice versa and the exigencies of every day life in rural Egypt can hardly be compared to those of an English town. It is also evident that the meaning of some items is totally different to the Egyptian respondents. Islamic philosophy encourages the perception of troubles as tests from God of the strength of one's faith - as one respondent expressed it: 'a problem or a trouble of today turns out to bring something good in the future'. There is thus a more general reluctance to regard anything as a 'problem' in the western sense and an even greater reluctance to make a public statement about it. As in other middle-eastern cultures, the public utterance of words relating to what are perceived as intimate issues causes offence. Most westerners have come to regard physical, social and mental status, however peculiar and personal as currency for open discussion. On a world basis, however, this is a minority view. Moreover, many of the preoccupations of westerners with anxiety, loneliness or insomnia have little meaning and no salience in other cultures.

The work of Whorf has influenced research concerned with the effects of linguistic relativity (Black, 1968). The idea that one can never really communicate with speakers of a language very different from one's own, because each language creates a different 'mind set' (Rosch, 1974) would, at first sight, seem to be partially confirmed here. However, as has been suggested, it might be more useful to ask, rather, in which domains communication between cultures is likely to be most inaccurate or inefficient (Dickson, Miyake and Takashi, 1977). It is clear that, problems of literal translation or functional equivalency aside, socio-emotional items are likely to cause the most trouble and items on what are perhaps more universal experiences, like pain, sleep and impaired physical mobility, the least.

A SPANISH VERSION OF THE SICKNESS IMPACT PROFILE

It may be that issues of cross-cultural equivalency are easier to solve where the cultures concerned are closer in language family and have at least some common background of history, mutual contact and daily experiences.

A description has been given of the development of a Spanish version of the Sickness Impact Profile (SIP) suitable for use with people of Mexican origin living in the USA (Gilson, Erickson, Chavez, Bobbitt, Bergner and Carter, 1980). The method of translation is based upon recommendations given by Pflanz (1973) for attaining item comparability. The method involved the production of four initial Chicano translations of the SIP by bilinguals. Each of these versions was back translated into English and compared to the original items by monolingual English raters. Combined ratings were used to choose the most acceptable translation. If disagreements between raters could not be resolved, the items were taken to a conference of the research team and the translators. Items which could not be resolved were eventually omitted from the final Chicano version.

The ensuing instrument was then tested for equivalence of response to the English and Spanish versions by giving it to bilingual persons likely to have comparatively high scores, (in fact, they were patients recently discharged from hospital). The English and Spanish versions were administered to each of 31 patients in a counterbalanced design with a 'short' (unspecified) interval between the two administrations and produced a high degree of agreement.

Rescaling of the items was also carried out in order to allow for differences in the severity with which some conditions might be viewed by Chicanos. However, equivalence of severity ratings was judged to be present and no changes in scale values were deemed necessary.

The methodology underlying this development and translation is exceptionally good, but reservations must be expressed concerning the low numbers of respondents involved, only 31 for the comparison of the English and Spanish version and 29 for the testing of the scale values. However, the number of suitable subjects available was probably small also, since the requirements for such a task are not solely that a person be reasonably fluent in two languages, but that he or she is likely to be suffering from a fairly severe condition, in order that the number of items affirmed is high enough to achieve the purpose of the exercise.

Deyo (1984) has criticised the development and use of the Chicano version of the SIP on the grounds that the validity of the items when used with Hispanics may be influenced by the fact that many of them are older and less well educated than either bilinguals or native Americans. Moreover, the seriousness with which they regard such a questionnaire may be low because of their lack of familiarity with the form, spirit, intent and assumptions of questionnaire administration and their lack of acculturation to the 'survey society'.

A SPANISH VERSION OF THE NOTTINGHAM HEALTH PROFILE

Similar criticisms may apply to the production of a Spanish version of the NHP. The Spanish speaking samples used were, in this case, of Cuban and Puerto Rican origin. However, they were generally well educated and living in or close to New York City, thus constituting a highly selected sample of the Spanish-speaking population of the USA.

A group of nine people bilingual in Spanish and English were recruited by personal contact and word of mouth. Five were Cuban and four were from Puerto Rico. They were asked, separately, to translate the instructions and items into their closest Spanish equivalents. Fortunately, differences between Cuban and Puerto Rican Spanish lie more in pronunciation than wording. This produced nine somewhat different versions. The items on physical mobility, pain and sleep produced the greatest agreement and emotional reactions the least.

Panel discussions were then held to attempt resolutions. It was decided that functional equivalence was preferable to literal translation - thus 'things are getting me down' became eventually 'las cosas me bajan el animo', literally, 'things are lowering my spirit'. 'The days seem to drag' became 'las dias paracen transcurrir lenta y pesadamente', literally, 'the days seem to go by slowly and heavily'.

Agreement was eventually reached on the wording of the instructions and all the items.

In order to test the equivalence of items in English and Spanish it was necessary, as in the Gilson et al. study, to contact individuals bilingual in these languages who might also be expected to have relatively poor perceived health and thus achieve fairly high scores on the Profile.

Eventually, subjects were contacted at a municipal clinic in Harlem, New York, and interviewed by a bilingual assistant, to assess their knowledge of both languages and to elicit their co-operation in the study. It proved impossible to obtain any kind of representative sample in this way, because many of the older patients (who were primarily female) did not speak English well enough to be suitable and many of the younger men did not wish to participate. (Harlem houses a high proportion of illegal immigrants, who, for obvious reasons, do not wish to reveal their name or address, or become involved with anything 'official'.). Over a period of five weeks 42 bilinguals from Cuba, Puerto Rico, Mexico and Venezuala were recruited, 31 of these were women aged 18 to 47 and 21 were males aged 29 to 52. The group were divided at random into two. Half were sent, by mail, an English profile, the other half the Spanish version. Thirty-eight profiles were returned, 20 Spanish and 18 English. Three weeks later the respondents were sent a further questionnaire in the other language. All 38 were returned.

Correlation coefficients showed adequate relationships between the scores in each language on both Part I and Part II.

It was thus concluded that this version in Spanish has face and content validity and has achieved equivalency with the English version, but that its overall validity and reliability may be severely restricted by the bias inherent in the samples used. It is currently being used as one of a set of outcome measures in a drug trial in USA. The resulting data may help in addressing these problems.

This version is now being considered for use in Spain where it will need to undergo further revision.

A NORTH AMERICAN VERSION OF THE NOTTINGHAM HEALTH PROFILE

Winston Churchill described the English and the Americans as two people separated by a common language. Disregarding this warning, requests to use the NHP in the United States led to the development of a version more acceptable to North Americans.

The Nottingham health Profile was given to a selected sample of 59 people living in New York and New Jersey. The subjects were broadly represent-ative of all socio-economic classes, except the very poorest and consisted of individuals who were at least second generation American. Subjects were asked to scrutinise the items and instructions for compatibility with American expression. There was surprisingly high agreement and very few suggestions for change. The term 'tick' in the instructions was changed to 'check', 'tablets' became 'pills'; 'I'm finding it hard to get on with people' was changed to 'get along with people'. Items which gave rise to disagreement were discussed in a group meeting consisting of researcher, student team and four panel members. A version of the NHP incorporating the changes was then distributed to patients attending a clinic at a dental hospital in New Jersey. In general, these patients represented middle to very low income groups. Profiles were issued at morning and afternoon clinics over a period of two months yielding an eventual sample of 527 persons in the age range 19-76 years, with 326 females and 201 males. Persons whose first language was not English were omitted. Patients were also asked about present minor and major illnesses and to give a rating of their health on a continuum from very good to very poor. Distribution of scores by age and sex was compared with that of British samples and found to follow a similar pattern with no significant differences. Scores also correlated highly with health ratings and the presence of diagnosed illness.

It was, therefore, concluded that the Nottingham Health Profile was suitable for use with samples of the North American population, although it should be borne in mind that the population is quite heterogeneous and the inhabitants of New York and New Jersey may differ a great deal from those of, say, Ohio, Tennessee or Wisconsin.

Due to lack of resources it was not possible to retest the weighting of items for the American or Spanish versions of the NHP. For the North American version this may not be so important since roughly equal distributions of scores to those found in Britain were obtained. However, for the Spanish version the current weightings may not be appropriate, although results from the Chicano version of the SIP seem to indicate a certain amount of cultural agreement on severity. Nevertheless, it would be recommended that this version should not be used without a preliminary check of the weightings. Nor have either of these versions been comprehensively tested so far for criterion validity or reliability.

Plans have been made to produce a fully validated French version of the NHP and to address systematically the methodological problems involved in such an enterprise.

CONCLUSIONS

Cross-cultural research and the use of health indicators in countries other than those in which they were developed requires a sound understanding of ethnomedicine, methodology and health services in the culture or cultures in question. Pflanz (1976) has listed several factors which must be taken into account.

1. The idiosyncracies of the particular official health system, for example tendencies to under- or over-counting.
2. The capacity of the system to ascertain, define and record particular diseases and disorders.
3. Tendencies to conceal 'unwanted' events, for example, outbreaks of cholera, suicides, abortions; biases and peculiarities in diagnosis.
4. Health behaviour and illness behaviour as culturally defined and sanctioned.
5. Advantages, disadvantages and manifestations of the sick role.
6. Different concepts of health and illness and their effects on utilisation of both traditional and western-style healers.

In non-industrialised countries there is obviously a need to produce means of identifying need and describing health problems that can be used by people with little or no medical training. Lay classifications as suggested by WHO (1978) and the development of instruments similar to the NHP, but appropriate to the culture, may be part of the answer. The measurement of health in a manner understandable to the public is also a priority. For this reason disability assessment should also be useful and field tests of questionnaires are at present being conducted by WHO using standard and cross-culturally comparable criteria of disability (Kohn and White, 1976).

It may well prove to be the case that the more 'subjective' or based upon perceived need the indicator, the more efficient and appropriate it would be to develop indicators in and for that culture specifically. The measurement of health status should derive its parameters from the most pressing needs of the citizenry of the country in question rather than being based upon culturally and perhaps medically irrelevant values.

REFERENCES

Aleyni, O. and Olayinka, A. (1978) 'An Evaluation of a Special Type of Vital Statistics Registration System in a Rural Area of Nigeria', Int J Epidemiol, 8, 61-68

Berger, P. and Luckmann, T. (1967) The Social Construction of Reality, Doubleday, New York

Bice, T.W. and Kalimo, E. (1971) Comparisons of Health-Related Attitudes - a Cross-National Factor Analytic Study', Soc Sci Med, 5, 283-318

Black, M. (1968) Linguistic Relativity: 'The Views of Benjamin Lee Whorf', in R. Manners and D. Kaplan (eds.), Theory in Anthropology: A Sourcebook, Aldine Atheron, Chicago, pp. 432-437

Blom, D.H.J. (1981) 'Objective Indices of Health in W. Zambia', Soc Sci Med, 15B, 395-398

Chance, N.A. (1962) 'Conceptual and Methodological Problems in Cross-Cultural Health Research', Am J Pub Hlth, 52, 410-417

Deyo, R.A. (1984) 'Pitfalls in Measuring the Health Status of Mexican Americans. Comparative Validity of the English and Spanish Sickness Impact Profile', Am J Pub Hlth, 74, 569-573

Dickson, W.P., Miyake, N.T. and Takashi, M. (1977) 'Referential Reltivity-Cultural Boundaries of Analytic and Metaphoric Communication', Cognition, 5, 215-233

Eyton, J. and Neuwirth, G. (1984) 'Cross-Cultural Validity: Ethnocentricity in Health Studies with Special Reference to the Vietnamese', Soc Sci Med, 18, 447-453

Frake, C.O. (1961) 'The Diagnosis of Disease among the Subanun of Mindanao', Amer Anthropologist, 63, 113-132

Gilson, B.S. Erickson, D. Chavez, C.T. Bobbitt, R.A. Bergner, M. and Carter, W.B. (1980) 'A Chicano Version of the Sickness Impact Profile (SIP)', Cult Med Psychiat, 4, 137-150

Harwood, A. (1970) Witchcraft, Sorcery and Social Categories among the Safwa, Oxford University Press, Oxford

Hsu, F.L.K. (1979) Psychosocial Homogeneities and Jen: Conceptual Tools for Advancing Psychological Anthropology', Amer Anthropologist, 73, 23-44

Kleinman, A., Eisenberg, L. and Good, B. (1978) 'Culture, Illness and Care. Clinical Lessons from Anthropologic and Cross-Cultural Research' Annals of Int Med, 88, 251-258

Kohn, R. and White, K.L. (eds.), (1976) Health Care: An International Study, Oxford University Press, London

Leff, J. (1977) 'The Cross-Cultural Study of Emotions', Culture, Medicine and Psychiatry, 1, 317-350

Lewis, G. (1975) Knowledge of Illness in Sepik Society, Athlone Press, London

Matesanz, A. (1974) 'The Psychometrically Sound Personality Questionnaire and its Adaptation into Other Languages', Revista de Psicologia General y Aplicada, 29, 1067-1085

Mitchell, R.E. (1968) 'Survey Materials Collected in the Developing Countries: Obstacles to Comparisons', in R. Rokkan (ed.), Comparative Research Across Cultures and Nations, Moulton, Paris, The Hague, pp. 176-205

Murnaghan, J. (1981) 'Health Indicators and Information Sytems for the Year 2000', Ann Rev Pub Hlth, 2, 299-362

Pflanz, M. (1973) Allgemeine Epidemiologie, Thieme, Stuttgart

Pflanz, M. (1976) 'Problems and Methods in Cross National Comparisons of Diagnoses and Diseases', in M. Pflanz and E. Schach (eds.), Cross National Sociomedical Research: Concepts, Methods and Practice, Thieme, Stuttgart, pp. 60-68

Racy, J. (1980) 'Somatization in Saudi Women: A Therapeutic Challenge', Brit J Psychiat, 137, 212-218

Rosch, E. (1974) 'Linguistic Relativity' in A. Silverstein (ed.), Human Communication - Theoretical Explorations, Wiley and Sons, New York

United Nations, (1972) Demographic Yearbook

1971, United Nations, New York

Vignes, J. and Hall, R. (1979) 'Adjustment of a Group of Vietnamese People to the USA, _Amer J Psychiat_, 136, 442-451

Werner, O. and Campbell, D. (1970) 'Translating, Working through Interpreters, and the Problem of Decentering' in R. Narrol and R. Cohen (eds.), _A Handbook of Method in Cultural Anthropology_, New York American Museum of Natural History, New York, pp. 398-420

World Health Organisation, (1978) _Lay Reporting of Health Information_, UNWHO, Geneva

Chapter 9.

USE AND ABUSE OF HEALTH INDICATORS

The approval by the 34th World health Assembly of twelve global indicators for the monitoring and evaluation of health strategies implies a commitment by member countries to their use (World Health Organisation, 1981a). In addition, regional indicators adapted to the needs of the areas concerned have been recommended and each country has been urged to adopt national indicators relevant to its special priorities (World Health Organiation, (1981b).

The importance of gathering information vital to learning about the health status and health needs of the world's citizens cannot be over-stated. Even more crucial is an understanding of the causes of the patterning of those needs across nations, populations and communities. Most important of all is that the needs should be addressed and met.

The development and use of a health indicator is not an end in itself. In some cases it seems that the soliciting of information by sophisticated means is in danger of becoming a substitute for tackling the problem. In the same way as statistical analysis is unnecessary when the figures are so extreme as to be unequivocal in meaning, so there is little point in expending time, resources and money on the exact delineation of issues that are self-evident and in the correction of which the resources would have been better spent. Traditional epidemiology has been criticised for reinforcing a 'positivist' approach to health care, which, although it has descriptive value, fails to tackle the underlying implications of its findings and ignores the implicit value system that it endorses - that a disease or health problem is largely, if not wholly, a biological phenomenon independent of the nature of the society within which it occurs and

225

where the subjective aspects of experience have no role (Paterson, 1981). It would be a great pity if the health indicators 'movement' became mere window dressing rather than an impetus for change in health care policies.

HEALTH INDICATORS IN PRIORITY SETTING

As we have already seen expenditure on health services as a percentage of the Gross National Product has been steadily increasing, although less so in Great Britain than in most other countries. There are several reasons for this increase but one of the primary factors is the existence of unnecessary and inappropriate services. It is notoriously difficult to link resources spent with benefits achieved, in terms of improved health, particularly when the traditional indicators such as mortality rates are used (Maxwell, 1974). From the consumer's perspective, it is care, cure and prevention which justify the continuing expense of the medical and health services establishment. In countries where medical and health care are coming to be focused in the area of chronic disorders the ultimate assessment of effective care can be made only by the patient. However, as Kelman (1975) has pointed out, the meaning that is given to health and the way in which it is assessed has implications for priorities and policies. Where a functional approach is adopted then the success of health strategies will be defined in terms of capacity for fulfilling those roles and tasks legitimised by the socialisation process. If, however, the focus is on experiential health, other values such as the development of human potential, freedom from adverse social demands and feelings of well-being will be emphasised. These, of course, are political decisions dependent upon the orientation of governments. The point is that the existence of health indicators and their use are not issues outside a political framework and do not necessarily imply some 'objective' approach to priority setting. This is the case whether the focus is on worldwide, national, local or clinical decision making.

For example, hitherto, decisions about who should receive which forms of care and in what form have been based upon medical opinion, customary usage or the traditional outcome measures supplemented by expediency. It remains to be seen how influential subjective measures such as the NHP can be in the decision making process. With long waiting lists for, say, hip replacements, priority might be given to those with the worst clinical picture, or to those who report the most distress, or to those who are judged most likely to benefit from the operation. The weight given to scores on a measure of perceived health problems will surely still depend upon the perspective of the orthopaedic surgeon and how far he is prepared to take them into account. What if they contradict his clinical judgement? The best outcome would be some trade-off between the two aspects with one type of indicator complementing the other, but this might be too much to expect given the long primacy of medical opinion.

At community level the use of small area analysis, for example, using postal code sectors, would allow the linking of data from instruments like the NHP to a variety of social indicators and to the use of health services. Most of the work on social deprivation and health risk points to a wide variation in the health experiences of sub-groups within deprived populations. Evidence in the Black Report (Department of Health and Social Security, 1980) shows that, although differences in health status are reflected in rates of incidence and prevalence and although health problems of most kinds are more numerous in the lower socio-economic groups, the occurrence of problems within these groups as a whole is still relatively uncommon. There is, thus, a need to identify sub-groups within generally disadvantaged populations in order to pinpoint those in greatest need. The closer delineation of pockets of need could facilitate the optimum distribution of resources. Again, however, the acceptability of the indicator and the imp- lications of the findings will be prime factors in whether or not changes in policy are implemented and action taken. After all, it has been known for several hundred years that the poor get sick more than their wealthier compatriots and though much research has been carried out, measurements taken and rhetoric expounded, very little has changed.

ETHICAL CONSIDERATIONS IN THE USE OF HEALTH MEASURES

In general there are two types of research carried out in the health service domain; therapeutic and non-therapeutic, although the boundaries of these are somewhat difficult to define. If the intent of the investigation is to evaluate the efficacy of a drug or surgical procedure then the aim is clearly therapeutic, not necessarily for the subjects taking part, but rather for future such patients. Where a questionnaire such as the NHP is used as part of clinical research, as was the case in the heart transplant programme, it is less obvious that there is a therapeutic objective. Non-therapeutic research is usually aimed at obtaining knowledge for a variety of purposes: testing theoretical models, as an aid to planning, to underpin policy decisions and so on.

The use of questionnaires is generally regarded as less intrusive than physical measures, but ethical considerations still arise with respect to three principal issues:

1. What is the justification for the use of this treatment and who will benefit from its use? Benefits may accrue to patients, for example, by improving treatment procedures or introducing alternative therapies such as counselling in cases of extreme distress. Society may benefit through the introduction of better ways of assessing need and meeting that need more efficiently. Or, and it may be sus-pected that this is usually the case, the researchers may be the sole beneficiaries, as they cut another notch in their totem of publications. Studies of the effects of health services research have, by and large, not been encouraging. It is very difficult to identify innovations and changes in procedures and policies ensuing from research findings (Lewis, 1977). Only rarely it seems have reports from health services research affected the minds of planners (Bice, 1980). However, it has ben argued that the main effect of research is less to initiate direct action than to alter the conceptual field of professionals and the public. Thus, Hofoss and Hjort (1981) maintain that the value of health service studies should be judged against conceptual development. If one accepts this view, then the use of socio-medical measures like the NHP can be justified. The idea that the public, whether receiving health care or not, should contribute their experiences and

evaluations is certainly gaining ground and the number of studies which now incorporate some form of self-report questionnaire into medical research is growing rapidly.

2. Can the research be designed and implemented in such a way that the results will justify the time, expense and intrusion into people's lives? It is a sad fact that although the utmost care is normally taken with the administration of medication, this is rarely the case when questionnaires are incorporated into clinical research. Questions may be answered under different conditions for each subject in the same study, conditions which may include a distracting physical environment.

    In community studies unless reasonable sampling procedures are used and the reliabiity and validity of the replies can be assessed and some information is obtainable on non-respondents, the results will be of dubious value.

3. Will the administration of this questionnaire pose any risk to the respondent? Filling in a questionnaire is not usually regarded as a hazardous undertaking, but it is possible that some form of harm might be done. For example, the fact that people are asked questions about their health may lead to hopes and raised expectations that something will be done to alleviate their distress, even if it has been explained to them that it is not the purpose of the exercise. On some questionnaires and as is the case with the NHP, the items could be regarded as depressing, focusing as they do on the negative aspects of experience. Statements such as 'I feel that life is not worth living' may be very upsetting for someone who is struggling to believe that it is. Conversely, the NHP does allow people to express the way they feel in a manner they understand, perhaps even leading them into thinking that they do not have so many problems as they previously imagined, especially in contrast to other people.

THE CONCEPT OF POSITIVE HEALTH

The statistics and indicators discussed in this book are quite clearly orientated towards medical services, designed, as they are, to measure aspects of disease, disability and distress in populations and selected groups. This focus on ill health as the legitimate concern of health and medical care has left a significant gap in our understanding of how people maintain good health even under quite adverse circumstances. Routine mortality statistics, hospital activities analysis or specially constructed instruments such as the General Household Survey or the NHP often assume the presence of health by the failure of respondents to affirm that they have health problems. Thus it has been inferred that people who do not use medical facilities or report illness on special surveys or otherwise come to the attention of those who gather information on such matters, are healthy. The inadequacy of such a situation is obvious, ignoring as it does factors influencing the use of services, gaps in the content of questionnaires and the existence of levels of unrecognised or unreported illness.

Very little is known about 'good health', how it is conceptualised by people, its distribution in populations and with what particular characteristics it is associated. The World Health Organisation's (1958) definition of health as physical, mental and social well-being, which was initially greeted with some scepticism, is now beginning to be seen as a description of a state which might, in some sense, be attainable by a majority of people, at least in the more affluent countries. The Department of Health and Social Security (1977) has shown interest in the idea that health services should contribute to well-being and an improved quality of life and Carter (1980) echoed this in his suggestion that the role of the Health Service should be that of moving people in the direction of good health, not simply away from disease and disability. It would seem that the movement towards an epidemiology of health, first recommended by Merrell and Reed in 1947 is gathering momentum. Although, as noted in chapter 3, there have been attempts to develop measures of well-being or to include items allowing responses indicative of good health, so far there are no satisfactory indicators of positive health. This is probably because of ignorance about what are the parameters of good health and what kinds of questions would be sufficiently sensitive and specific to elicit reliable and valid data. The experience of those who gathered the initial information from the interviews on which the items in the NHP were based, was that the paucity of language for expressing good health or well-being was such that it would be very difficult to construct a comprehensive set of items. Research has suggested that lay people do show some agreement on concepts of health and differentiate between ideas of 'good health', 'well-being' and 'fitness' (Herzlich, 1973; Pill and Stott, 1980; Williams, 1981; Hunt and Macleod, 1985). However, the problem is that 'good health' is both socially defined and individually perceived and is relative to other factors, particularly age and social role require-ments. Positive health in a seven year old boy will be different from its manifestations in a seventy year old woman. It would, therefore, be necessary to develop age-related norms if 'good health' were to be self-assessed. On the other hand, if a professional perspective were adopted positive health might be found to be rare indeed. There is obviously a great deal more conceptual and methodological work to do before there could be sufficiently reliable and valid data to enable the construction of a positive health indicator, even if there were more than verbal support for such an enterprise.

It may well be that this apparent move towards a concern with 'good health' is no more than the current rhetoric of various health agencies. Certainly, few resources are being devoted to its research or promotion. In addition, some writers have expressed anxiety that putting efforts into the identification of 'positive health' which has, at present, no relevance to current health policies, may detract from issues of more pressing importance whose amelioration is within the scope of contemporary practice (Bice, 1979).

THE NOTTINGHAM HEALTH PROFILE: RETROSPECT AND PROSPECT

The original rationale for the development of the NHP was to have an instrument which could be used as a population survey tool and contribute to:

1. The identification of groups in need of care.

2. Social policy, through helping to determine the allocation of resources.
3. Mass aspects of the evaluation of health and social services.
4. The identification of consumer concerns.
5. The theoretical understanding of the relationship between perception and pathology.

It seems appropriate to ask, at this stage, how far such an instrument has, or could fulfil these objectives.

The conceptual basis of the NHP was that it should reflect lay definitions of health; thus avoiding professional debates about appropriate concepts of health. However, the sobriquet 'health profile' is really misleading. It has become increasingly obvious that what the NHP measures cannot be delineated by any of the usual labels - health status, illness, disease, morbidity, functional capacity. It appears to relate rather to how people feel when they are experiencing various states of ill health, disability or discomfort, whether psychic or physical; hence the close association of the scores with chronic conditions, utilisation patterns and social circumstances, such as unemployment. It now appears to the authors that it is more useful to think of the NHP as a measure of distress, where this distress may be a consequence of pathological changes requiring medical and health services, but equally may be a result of adverse social and/or environmental occurrences or conditions.

Outcome measures for the evaluation of medical treatment and care have normally been of a kind presumed to reflect solely the medical aspects of the system of care. However, the validity of such measures has been rather low since many outcomes are related more to socio-economic factors and the general emotional state of the patient than to purely medical factors. In particular, the impact of health and medical services at the primary level is profoundly influenced by social, psychological and environmental conditions, such as income, housing and self-esteem. The principle value of the NHP is that it can identify levels of distress which may exist regardless of biological health status. It has shown for example, that medical intervention may cure the presenting problem, but do little to alleviate suffering of an existential kind. The NHP may, therefore, have a major role in the evaluation of service provision particularly when used in conjunction with a more clinically orientated indicator of health status. In this way, a more precise understanding of the effect of health services on 'well-being' that goes beyond mere functional capacity may be obtained.

The identification of groups in need of care is a feasible objective for the NHP as has been demonstrated in both clinical and community studies. Surveys at community level conducted in areas known to be characterised by an unusually high number of health problems can provide information about which residents in which particular locations are likely to have unmet needs. Linking these data to general practitioner records, referrals for consultations and hospital admissions should help in elucidating the role and extent of health services in addressing the 'career' of the patient. The major issue here is rather the nature of the care that is needed.

Writers such as Illich (1975), Carlson (1975) and Arney and Bergen (1984) have drawn attention to what is sometimes referred to as the 'medicalisation of the human condition'. This process may take various forms and appear sinister or humanitarian depending upon one's own set of values, but it is said to manifest itself in the tendency to bring fairly common human problems such as drunkenness, crime, infertility or obesity within the province of medicine or to make normal human events such as birth and death into medical issues. The repercussions of this are the conversion of moral dilemmas into technical problems to be treated from the armamentarium of medical technology; the transformation of natural experiences into tasks for medical management; the erosion of individual responsibility and the encouragement of the idea that almost any human experience which gives rise to distress can be conceptualised as a health or medical matter.

It is feasible that the development of certain types of indicator, including the Nottingham Health Profile, play a part in 'medicalisation' by giving the rubric of 'health' to forms of distress which are much more likely to be alleviated by socioeconomic and political reforms than by health or medical care. A good example of this is in the use of the NHP with inner city samples and in studies of social deprivation. The fact that the lower social classes report more problems and distress than the higher, especially on emotional reactions, sleep, energy and social isolation, is not necessarily a manifestation of health problems nor an indication that more health care is needed. At the end of a study of social inequalities and perceived health it was concluded that:

> The evidence produced here suggests that it is unlikely that a change in the allocation of health care resources would have more than a minor influence on inequalities in health. The alleviation of such distress as we have found goes far beyond a tinkering with the methods of delivering primary care. Indeed, efforts devoted to minor alterations in health care delivery may serve to distract people from the real nature of the problem. Remedial action would need to take the more radical form of providing a climate in which social and occupational aspirations had a greater chance of being fulfilled, with greater resources being allocated not to health care, but to those fundamental social and environmental reforms which would enhance well-being and ameliorate the cycle of deprivation.

(Hunt, McEwen and McKenna, 1985, p. 158.).

Clearly, it is important that the use of a health indicator to assess, let us say, unmet needs, does not lead inexorably to the conclusion that the root cause of those needs is a health problem and the best panacea is a dose of health services. It is, however, possible, that where it can be established that 'pockets' of distress exist special programmes could be established by, say, district or regional authorities, to address these in a way which involved an integrated approach by all the departments concerned - that is, for example, health, housing, environmental health, education and so on. Also it should not be forgotten that health and medical issues may be powerful political levers involving, as they do, emotive terms which arouse public sympathy more than do more mundane-sounding social needs. Thus there may be occasions when describing something as a health issue may be the best way to elicit remedial action. Where the cause of the distress clearly lies in the health status of the patient the identification of need for care can lead to the provision of counselling, social support, domiciliary and other services which are within the remit and capability of the health and social services.

A contribution to the mass evaluation of health

and social services seems, in retrospect, to have been pretentious and unrealistic. The fact that, in a random sample, the NHP yields a high number of zero scorers makes it unsuitable for such a large goal. On the other hand with selected groups it appears to be sensitive and reliable enough for the assessment of both process and outcome consequent upon specified interventions. The most useful applications of the NHP so far have been with socially disadvantaged groups and chronically ill patients where scores are relatively high and the significance of changes can be evaluated with confidence and comparisons made.

At the present time a contribution to social policy seems a remote prospect for such a modest instrument. However, studies past and in progress are increasing our knowledge of the effect of various local and institutional practices. With sufficient and consistent data it is possible that small changes in policy may occur.

The theoretical aspects of the relationship between perception and pathology have received little attention so far. Most uses of the NHP to date have been entirely practical, either involving the developmental tasks of the instrument itself or pragmatic aspects of survey and evaluative studies. There does, however, seem to be some promise in two areas. Links between social inequalities and levels of distress provide support for a theory of psychosocial vulnerability as a major contributor to ill health and differences in patterns of scores for patients with similar disorders may eventually contribute to a model of coping strategies. The collation of data from a large number of projects using the NHP would obviously help to elucidate some of these issues as well as consolidate the establishment of 'norms' for different groups. When giving permission for the use of the NHP by others, the authors have normally done so in exchange for a promise of the raw data. Alas, such promises have yet to be fulfilled.

The various shortcomings of the NHP as it stood at the end of the development period in 1981 have been described and are summarised in the Appendix. Since then two important optional amendments have been made.

Firstly, it was realised that Part II was not always a useful or unequivocal addition. For many groups, the elderly, unemployed, people on low incomes, the chronically disabled, several of the items did not apply. Moreover, it was often not clear whether the various activities were being affected by health problems <u>per se</u> or whether they were attributed to health problems <u>post hoc</u>. The aggregation of scores into percentages for groups produces a statistic of uncertain worth wherein certain factors may be confounded. Occasionally this may not matter, for example, if information is needed on how many people are restricted in some activity for whatever reason or where all items should be relevant to all respondents. However, when this is not the case it seems preferable to omit Part II altogether. Experiments putting Part II at the beginning of the questionnaire have been made, together with asking respondents to what they attribute any effects being experienced in the seven areas of daily life. At the moment it is not clear whether this has any more advantages than the original format.

Secondly, it was known that when the NHP was used as a postal questionnaire, the response rate was depressed by the number of zero scorers - that is, people who thought they had nothing to communicate were less inclined to return the questionnaire. A study is now in progress where 'dummy' items of a positive nature, for example, 'I sleep soundly at night', 'I am usually free of any pain', have been interspersed with the original items. This is currently yielding an 85 per cent response rate from a group selected by age and sex, but otherwise from a 'normal' population.

Currently, as far as is known, the NHP is being used in a study of patients on renal dialysis, a comparison of attenders and non-attenders at a breast breast screening clinic, in drug trials, as a measure of quality of life in patients suffering from cardio-vascular disease, in assessments of interventions with the elderly, in community surveys, in studies of unemployment, in an invest-igation into the effects of damp and overcrowded housing and in evaluations of various aspects of occupational health. It is also undergoing translations and revisions to make it suitable for use in Spain, Sweden and France. Should these adaptations prove successful there is potential for cross-cultural comparisons in perceptions of distress in relation to social, health and medical services and the process and and outcome of interventions.

Measures of self-perceived health have some special characteristics of particular relevance to present day debates on the provision of health services:

1.   They are determined by the lay public rather than by medical and nosological criteria. Since fifty percent of people consulting a doctor cannot be classified by the International Classification of Diseases (White, 1974) this is an important consideration.

2.   They are related to perceived distress and/or its impact on function and are, therefore, more closely tied to behaviour than are medical diagnoses. They thus have potential for picking up individuals missed by the health services.

3.   They can assess levels of distress associated with the same medical condition and thus identify priority groups within a diagnostic category.

4.   They are capable of identifying types of perceived ill health within populations and may provide pointers to social problems and emotional disability as well as physical conditions.

5.   They can be used to evaluate health and medical services in respect of how they affect the way people feel, in distinction to, say, surgical criteria.

6.   They can help clarify the processes which mediate the connection between 'subjective' and 'objective' health.

7.   They are readily understood by and are acceptable to the general public and, to the extent that allocation of resources should reflect the views and needs of society, have potential for greater equity of provision relative to need.

8.   Perceptions as to what constitutes illness and health and when professional help should be sought differ according to social grouping and culture. Self-report measures which refer to rather specific experiences have a relatively low chance of being interpreted in more than one way. Thus it is possible to compare groups having the same or similar levels of perceived distress in terms of their utilisation of services, diagnosis, social or physical environment and health-related behaviour.

CONCLUSION

The construction and the dimensions of a health indicator are, as pointed out by Culyer (1978), partly a question of values and partly a technical undertaking. The Nottingham Health Profile represents an attempt to reflect the values of the consumers of health services without sacrificing the scientific methodology which would make it acceptable to professional groups. It may not be the best or the last of its type, but we hope it may play some role in establishing a means of moving health and medical care towards a more co-operative enterprise between professionals and public and in drawing attention to those aspects of the social structure which are implicated in the aetiology of distress.

REFERENCES

Arney, W.R. and Bergen, B.J. (1984) Medicine and the Management of Living, University of Chicago Press, Chicago

Bice, T.W. (1979) 'Comments on Health Indicators: Methodological Perspectives' in J. Elinson and A. Siegmann (eds.), Socio-Medical Health Indicators, Baywood, Farmingdale, New York, pp. 185-195

Bice, T.W. (1980) 'Social Science and Health Services Research: Contributors to Public Policy', Milb Mem Fd Quart, 2, 173-186

Carlson, R. (1975) The End of Medicine, Wiley Interscience, New York

Carter, C. (1980) 'The Purposes of Welfare Services' in Discussing the Welfare State, Discussion Paper No. 1, Policy Studies Institute, London, pp. 1-22

Culyer, A.J. (1978) 'Need, Values and Health Service Measurment' in A.J. Culyer and K.S. Wright (eds.), Economic Aspects of Health Services, Martin Robertson, York

Department of Health and Social Security (1977) Prevention and Health, Cmnd 7047, HMSO, London

Department of Health and Social Security (1980) Inequalities in Health: Report of a Research Working Group, (The Black Report), HMSO, London

Herzlich, C. (1973) Health and Illness: A Social Psychological Approach, Academic Press, New Jersey

Hofoss, D. and Hjort, P.F. (1981) 'The Relationship between Action and Research in Health Policy', Soc Sci Med, 15A, 371-375

Hunt, S.M. and McEwen, J. (1980) 'The Development of a Subjective Health Indicator', Sociol Hlth Illness, 2, 231-246

Hunt, S.M. McEwen, J. and McKenna, S. (1985) 'Social Inequalities and Perceived Health', Effective Health Care, 2, 151-160

Hunt, S.M. and Macleod, M. (1985) 'Health and Behavioural Change: Some Lay Perspectives', Community Medicine, (under editorial consideration)

Illich, I. (1975) Medical Nemesis: The Expropriation of Health, Calder and Boyars, London

Kelman, S. (1975) 'The Social Nature of the Definition Problem in Health', Int J Hlth Serv, 5, 625-642

Lewis, C.E. (1977) 'Health Services Research and Innovations in Health Care Delivery', New Eng J Med, 19, 1073-1077

Maxwell, R. (1974) Health Care: The Growing Dilemma, McKinsey, New York

Merrell, M. and Reed, L.J. (1947) 'The Epidemiology of Health' in I. Galdston (ed.), Social Medicine: Its Derivatives and Objectives, New York Academy of Medicine Institute of Social Medicine, The Commonwealth Fund, New York

Paterson, K. (1981) 'Theoretical Perspectives in Epidemiology - A Critical Appraisal', Radical Comm Med, 8, 21-29

Pill, R. and Stott, N. (1982) 'Concepts of Illness Causality and Responsibility: Some Preliminary Data from a Sample of Working Class Mothers', Soc Sci Med, 16, 43-52

White, K. (1974) 'Contemporary Epidemiology', Int J Epidemiol, 3, 140-163

World Health Organisation (1958) The First Ten Years of the World Health Organisation, WHO, Geneva

World Health Organisation (1981a) Global Strategy for Health for All by the Year 2000, Health for All, Series, 3, WHO, Geneva

World Health Organisation (1981b) Development of Indicators for Monitoring Progress towards Health for All by the Year 2000, Health for All, Series, 4, WHO, Geneva

APPENDIX

NOTTINGHAM HEALTH PROFILE

BEFORE YOU START

Please be sure to read the instructions

LISTED BELOW ARE SOME PROBLEMS PEOPLE MAY HAVE IN
THEIR DAILY LIFE.
LOOK DOWN THE LIST AND PUT A TICK IN THE BOX
UNDER <u>YES</u> FOR ANY PROBLEM YOU HAVE AT THE MOMENT.
TICK THE BOX UNDER <u>NO</u> FOR ANY PROBLEM YOU DO NOT
HAVE.

<u>PLEASE ANSWER EVERY QUESTION</u>. IF YOU ARE NOT SURE
WHETHER TO SAY YES OR NO, TICK WHICHEVER ANSWER YOU
THINK IS <u>MORE TRUE</u> AT THE MOMENT.

	YES	NO
I'm tired all the time	☐	☐
I have pain at night	☐	☐
Things are getting me down	☐	☐

	YES	NO
I have unbearable pain	☐	☐
I take tablets to help me sleep	☐	☐
I've forgotten what it's like to enjoy myself	☐	☐

	YES	NO
I'm feeling on edge	☐	☐
I find it painful to change position	☐	☐
I feel lonely	☐	☐

	YES	NO
I can only walk about indoors	☐	☐
I find it hard to bend	☐	☐
Everything is an effort	☐	☐

	YES	NO
I'm waking up in the early hours of the morning	☐	☐
I'm unable to walk at all	☐	☐
I'm finding it hard to make contact with people	☐	☐

	YES	NO
The days seem to drag	☐	☐
I have trouble getting up and down stairs or steps	☐	☐
I find it hard to reach for things	☐	☐

REMEMBER IF YOU ARE NOT SURE WHETHER TO
ANSWER YES OR NO TO A PROBLEM, TICK
WHICHEVER ANSWER YOU THINK IS <u>MORE TRUE</u>
AT THE MOMENT.

	YES	NO
I'm in pain when I walk	☐	☐
I lose my temper easily these days	☐	☐
I feel there is nobody I am close to	☐	☐

	YES	NO
I lie awake for most of the night	☐	☐
I feel as if I'm losing control	☐	☐
I'm in pain when I'm standing	☐	☐

243

3.

	YES	NO
I find it hard to dress myself	☐	☐
I soon run out of energy	☐	☐
I find it hard to stand for long (eg at the kitchen sink, waiting for a bus)	☐	☐

	YES	NO
I'm in constant pain	☐	☐
It takes me a long time to get to sleep	☐	☐
I feel I am a burden to people	☐	☐

	YES	NO
Worry is keeping me awake at night	☐	☐
I feel that life is not worth living	☐	☐
I sleep badly at night	☐	☐

	YES	NO
I'm finding it hard to get on with people	☐	☐
I need help to walk about outside (eg a walking aid or someone to support me)	☐	☐
I'm in pain when going up and down stairs or steps	☐	☐

	YES	NO
I wake up feeling depressed	☐	☐
I'm in pain when I'm sitting	☐	☐

NOW WE WOULD LIKE YOU TO THINK ABOUT THE
ACTIVITIES IN YOUR LIFE WHICH MAY BE
AFFECTED BY HEALTH PROBLEMS.

IN THE LIST BELOW, TICK YES FOR EACH ACTIVITY IN
YOUR LIFE WHICH IS BEING AFFECTED BY YOUR STATE OF
HEALTH. TICK NO FOR EACH ACTIVITY WHICH IS NOT
BEING AFFECTED, OR WHICH DOES NOT APPLY TO YOU.

Is your present state of health causing
problems with your ...   YES   NO

JOB OF WORK   ☐   ☐
(That is, paid employment)

LOOKING AFTER THE HOME   ☐   ☐
(Examples: cleaning & cooking, repairs
 odd jobs around the home etc)

SOCIAL LIFE   ☐   ☐
(Examples: going out, seeing friends,
 going to the pub etc)

HOME LIFE   ☐   ☐
(That is: relationships with other
 people in your home)

SEX LIFE   ☐   ☐

INTERESTS AND HOBBIES   ☐   ☐
(Examples: sports, arts and crafts,
 do-it-yourself etc)

HOLIDAYS   ☐   ☐
(Examples: summer or winter holidays,
 weekends away etc)

NOW GO BACK TO PAGE 1 AND MAKE SURE
YOU HAVE ANSWERED YES OR NO TO EVERY
QUESTION ON ALL THE PAGES

The Nottingham
Health Profile

M A N U A L

The Nottingham Health Profile is a two-part self-administered questionnaire designed to measure perceived health problems and the extent to which such problems affect normal activities.

It is appropriate for use in the following ways:

1. For evaluation of medical/social interventions, in pre-test, post-test designs.
2. As an outcome measure for group comparisons.
3. As a survey tool with specified groups, e.g. the elderly, the chronically ill.
4. As an adjunct to clinical interviews.

The Nottingham Health Profile is equally efficient administered by an interviewer or sent by post. It can be used with populations aged 16 years and upwards and requires a minimum reading age of 10 years.

Copyright is held on the NHP in Great Britain and USA by Hunt, McEwen and McKenna and permission to use it should be sought from one of the authors.

DEVELOPMENT OF THE PROFILE

Work began on the construction of the NHP in September 1975 and was completed by December 1981.

Early work was devoted to collecting statements from the general public which described the typical effects of ill-health. The effects encompassed social, psychological, behavioural and physical functioning e.g. 'I am sleeping badly', 'I've lost interest in sex', 'I can't keep my mind on my work', 'I find it hard to walk upstairs'.

An initial collection of 2,200 statements enabled key concepts to be identified. Statements were then drawn which exemplified those concepts. After eliminating those which were redundant, ambiguous, esoteric, or required too high a reading age, a total of 138 statements were left.

Combinations of the remaining statements were used in a number of pilot and major studies between 1976 and 1978. These studies carried out on several different populations enabled the number of statements to be refined and further reduced to 82.

By relating scores on the questionnaire to medical information and independent assessments of patients' well-being, as well as other standardised measures, it was found that the items were reliable and valid in distinguishing between different degrees of disability and sensitive to changes over time. In addition they were able to distinguish between physical and mental disorders (Martini, C.J.M. and McDowell, I. 1976; McDowell, I. and Martini, C.J.M. 1976; Martini, C.J.M. and McDowell, I. 1977; McDowell, I. Martini, C.M.J. and Waugh, W. 1978).

A closer look was then taken at the statements in order to develop the questionnaire in a manner which would make it suitable for inclusion in a population survey.

The existing statements were, therefore, re-tested and analysed using the following criteria for selection:

1. There should be no negative expressions.
2. Statements should be easy to answer, easy to understand and unambiguous.
3. Statements should be answerable by 'yes' or 'no'.
4. Language used should conform to standards of a minimum reading age.

Each item was the subject of discussion by the research team and once it was found to have met the above criteria, it was tested on a sample of patients and non-patients for clarity of meaning, consensus of meaning and ease of answering. Those statements which passed these tests were retained.

Statements were categorised into six areas: physical mobility, pain, sleep, energy, emotional reactions and social isolation.

A respondent is required to indicate 'yes' or 'no' according to whether the statement applies to him or her 'in general at the present time'. This comprises Part I of the NHP.

The content of the Part II was gained from analysis of interviews with patients. It was found that, overall, seven areas of daily life were most often mentioned as being affected by health – these were work, looking after the home, social life, home life, sex life, interests and hobbies and holidays.

VALIDATION STUDIES

The NHP has been tested for face, content and criterion validity and has been found to be a highly satisfactory measure of subjective health status, in the physical, social and emotional domains; and to be a useful guide to the extent by which health problems restrict normal physical and social activities.

Testing has taken place with the following groups:

1. Four groups of elderly people (over 65).

   i) 41 people participating in a research programme on physical exercise who could be described as 'fit' on the basis of their exercise heart rate.
   ii) A sample of 19 patients drawn from the records of a general practitioner who had no known illness or disability and who had not contacted a doctor for at least two months prior to the study.
   iii) 49 people with a variety of health and social problems, attending a luncheon club run by the social services.
   iv) 54 chronically ill patients drawn from GP records and divided into two groups.

   Results showed that NHP scores effectively differentiated between the 'well' groups (i and ii) and 'ill' groups (iii and iv). The study also indicated that the content of the statements was understood by and acceptable to elderly persons (Hunt, S.M. McKenna, S.P. McEwen, J. Backett, E.M. Williams, J. and Papp, E. 1980).

2. 352 persons drawn at random from GP
    records and divided into two groups:

    i) Consulters, i.e. persons who had
        consulted the general practitioner
        more than three times in the
        previous six month period.
    ii) Non-consulters, i.e. persons who
        had not consulted the doctor at
        all in the same six month period.

    Controlling for age, sex and consultation
    rate, the NHP scores showed significant
    differences between the scores of the
    groups on all sections. Scores were also
    associated with reported absence from work
    through ill health (Hunt, S.M. McKenna,
    S.P. McEwen, J. Williams, J. and Papp, E.
    1981).

3. 158 firemen representing a 'fit' sample.
    NHP scores were very low for the group
    as a whole but some individuals achieved
    very high scores on energy, sleep and
    emotional reactions (McKenna, S.P. Hunt,
    S.M. McEwen, J. Williams, J. and Papp, E.
    1980).

4. 113 mine rescue workers representing 'fit'
    workers. Scores were very low, with 79
    per cent of the sample reporting no
    problems at all (McKenna, S.P. Hunt, S.M.
    and McEwen, J. 1981).

5. 80 pregnant women who were administered
    the NHP at three stages during their
    pregnancy - 18, 27 and 37 weeks. Results
    showed the NHP to be sensitive to changes
    occurring during pregnancy (Backett, E.M.
    McEwen, J. and Hunt, S.M. 1981).

6. 93 patients with peripheral vascular
    disease who were attending an outpatient
    clinic. Scores reflected the high number
    of problems experienced by these patients
    especially in the areas of pain, sleep
    disturbance and physical mobility (Hunt,
    S.M. McEwen, J. McKenna, S.P. and Pope, C.
    1984).

7. 141 patients attending a fracture clinic
    and an equal number of control subjects.
    NHP scores were obtained from patients and
    controls at a point in time soon after the
    fracture occurred and again eight weeks
    later. Scores were sensitive to changes

in perceived health concomitant with the healing of the fracture (McKenna, S.P. McEwen, J. Hunt, S.M. and Papp, E. 1984).

8. 157 patients attending an out-patient clinic for non-acute complaints such as haemorrhoids, hernias, varicose veins, ulcers etc. Results showed the patients as a whole to have a perceived health status below that of people who consider themselves to be well (Hunt, S.M. McEwen, J. McKenna, S.P. and Pope, C. 1984).

9. A random sample of 2173 people drawn from a group general practice in the Nottingham area. Results showed significant differences in scores between social classes, age groups and sexes (Hunt, S.M. McEwen, J. and McKenna, S.P. 1985).

10. A sample of 1756 people at work drawn from a large industrial organisation in the Nottingham area. Results showed differences in scores between social classes age groups and sexes, similar to the general practice sample (McEwen, J. Lowe, D. Hunt, S.M. and McKenna, S.P. 1985).

These studies have established the validity of the NHP for use with a wide range of people and age groups.

RELIABILITY STUDIES

Two studies have been carried out to establish the reliability of NHP scores in terms of their consistency over time. Both studies utilised the test, re-test technique.

Since a high percentage of negative responses would give a spurious consistency, it was necessary to use groups of people who could be expected to be high scorers.

1. 58 patients with osteoarthritis were selected for study, specifically those awaiting hip replacement operations. Each person was sent a NHP and covering letter by mail and a second questionnaire was sent four weeks later (Hunt, S.M. McKenna, S.P. and Williams, J. 1981). Reliability coefficients are shown in Tables 1 and 2.

2. 93 patients with peripheral vascular disease were given the questionnaire to

Table 1 Correlation coefficients on each section of
Part I (* p < .001) (Patients with Osteoarthrosis).

	Spearman's r	
Energy	0.77	*
Pain	0.79	*
Emotional reactions	0.80	*
Sleep	0.85	*
Social isolation	0.78	*
Physical mobility	0.85	*

Table 2 Correlation coefficients for statements on
Part II (*p < .001) (Patients with Osteoarthrosis)

	Cramer's C	
Work	0.86	*
Looking after the home	0.85	*
Social life	0.59	*
Home life	0.64	*
Sex life	0.84	*
Interests and hobbies	0.44	*
Holidays	0.71	*

complete and were sent a second one eight
weeks later (Hunt, S.M. McEwen, J.
McKenna, S.P. Backett, E.M. and Pope, C.
1982). Tables 3 and 4 show the reliability coefficients.

These two studies demonstrate the high level of
reliability of the NHP with groups suffering from
chronic illness.
It should be noted that certain changes in
perceived health may have occurred between the two
administrations of the questionnaire, consequently
reducing the correlation obtained. This is a
general problem with testing the reliability of a
sensitive indicator, since the greater the
sensitivity of the instrument to change, the lower
will be the consistency between administrations of
the instrument to the same group of people.

Table 3 Correlation coefficients on each section of Part I (*p < .001) (Patients with Peripheral Vascular Disease).

Energy	0.77	*
Pain	0.88	*
Emotional reactions	0.75	*
Sleep	0.85	*
Social isolation	0.77	*
Physical mobility	0.79	*

Table 4 Correlation coefficients for statements on Part II (*p< .001) (Patients with Peripheral Vascular Disease).

Work	0.55	*
Looking after the home	0.64	*
Social life	0.61	*
Home life	0.89	*
Sex life	0.85	*
Interests and hobbies	0.86	*
Holidays	0.72	*

ADMINISTRATION

The NHP was designed to be self-administered and very few problems will be encountered using it this way. It is also possible to read out the statements to individuals who have sight or reading problems. It can be administered by an interviewer either to an individual or on a group basis.

Studies in which the NHP has been sent through by post have yielded response rates between 68 per cent and 93 per cent. Its success as a postal questionnaire is highly dependent upon the population being sampled, appropriate preparatory discussions and the content and source of the covering letter.

SCORING

Responses are best coded 1 for 'yes' and 0 for 'no'. On Part I these can then be converted to the appropriate weights by computer programme and summed to give the total on each section.

The weights and computer codes are given in Table 5 and an example of computer conversion to weighted scores is given on pages 254-258. This format is suitable for analysis using the Statistical Package for the Social Sciences.

Part II is simply coded 1 for 'yes' and 0 for 'no'.

WEIGHTING OF STATEMENTS IN PART I

Since the various statements in each section vary in severity, they have been weighted by means of Thurstone's Method of Paired Comparisons.

The weights of the statements on each of the six sections total 100 which represents a situation where the respondent answers affirmatively all the statements in that section. Hence the higher the score on a section, the greater the perceived health problems in that area.

Table 5   Weighted scores for 'yes' responses on Part I.

STATEMENT	WEIGHT	CODE
I'm tired all the time	39.20	EN1
I have pain at night	12.91	P1
Things are getting me down	10.47	EM1
I have unbearable pain	19.74	P2
I take tablets to help me sleep	22.37	SL1
I've forgotten what it's like to enjoy myself	9.31	EM2
I'm feeling on edge	7.22	EM3
I find it painful to change position	9.99	P3
I feel lonely	22.01	SO1
I can only walk about indoors	11.54	PM1
I find it hard to bend	10.57	PM2
Everything is an effort	36.80	EN2
I'm waking up in the early hours of the morning	12.57	SL2
I'm unable to walk at all	21.30	PM3

Table 5 (cont): Weighted Scores for 'Yes' Responses
on Part I

STATEMENT	WEIGHT	CODE
I'm finding it hard to make contact with people	19.36	SO3
The days seem to drag	7.08	EM4
I have trouble getting up and down stairs or steps	10.79	PM4
I find it hard to reach for things	9.30	PM5
I'm in pain when I walk	11.22	P4
I lose my temper easily these days	9.76	EM5
I feel there is nobody I am close to	20.13	SO3
I lie awake for most of the night	27.26	SL3
I feel as if I'm losing control	13.99	EM6
I'm in pain when I'm standing	8.96	P5
I find it hard to dress myself	12.61	PM6
I soon run out of energy	24.00	EN3
I find it hard to stand for long (eg at the kitchen sink, waiting for a bus)	11.20	PM7
I'm in constant pain	20.86	P6
It takes me a long time to get to sleep	16.10	SL4
I feel I am a burden to people	22.53	SO4
Worry is keeping me awake at night	13.95	EM7
I feel that life is not worth living	16.21	EM8
I sleep badly at night	21.70	SL5
I'm finding it hard to get on with people	15.97	SO5
I need help to walk about outside (eg a walking aid or someone to support me)	12.69	PM8
I'm in pain when going up and down stairs or steps	5.83	P7
I wake up feeling depressed	12.01	EM9
I'm in pain when I'm sitting	10.49	P8

Table 6   Scoring for 'yes' responses on Part II

STATEMENT	SCORE FOR 'YES'
Is your present state of health causing problems with your ...	
Job of work (That is, paid employment)	1
Looking after the home (Examples; cleaning and cooking, repairs, odd jobs around the home etc)	1
Social life (Examples; going out, seeing friends, going to the pub etc)	1
Home life (That is, relationships with other people in your home)	1
Sex life	1
Interests and hobbies (Examples; sports, arts and crafts, do-it-yourself etc)	1
Holidays (Examples; summer or winter holidays, weekends away etc)	1

Coding of Part I Responses by Computer Programme (SPSS Format)

RECODE   EN1(1=39.2)/P1(1=12.91)/EM1(1=10.47
)/P2(1=19.74)/SL1(1=22.37)/EM2(1=
                 9.31)/EM3(1=7.22)P3(1=9.99)/SO1(1=
                 22.01)/ PM1(1=11.54)/PM2(1=10.57)/
                 EN2(1=36.8)/SL2(1=12.57)/PM3(1=21.3
)/ SO2(1=19.36)/EM4(1=7.08)/PM4(1=
                 10.79)/PM5(1=9.3)/P4(1=11.22)

RECODE   EM5(1=9.76)/SO3(1=20.13)/SL3/(1=27.
                 26)/EM6(1=13.99)/P5(1=8.96)/
                 PM6(1=12.61)/EN3(1=24)/PM7(1=11.2)/

Coding of Part I Responses by Computer Programme (cont)

```
                   P6(1=20.86)/SL4(1=16.1)/SO4(1=22.53
                   )/ EM7(1=13.95)/EM8(1=16.21)/SL5
                   (1=21.7)/SO5(1=15.97)/PM8(1=12.69)/
                   P7(1=5.83)/EM(1=12.01)/P8(1=10.49)
```

COMPUTE	TEN=EN1+EN2+EN3
COMPUTE	TP=P1+P2+P3+P4+P5+P7+P8
COMPUTE	TEM=EM1+EM2+EM3+EM4+EM5+EM6+EM7+EM8 + EM9
	TSL=SL1+SL2+SL3+SL4+SL5
COMPUTE	TSO=SO1+SO2+SO3+SO4+SO5
COMPUTE	TPM=PM1+PM2+PM3+PM4+PM5+PM6+PM7+PM8
COMPUTE	
MISSING VALUES	EN1 to P8(9)
ASSIGN MISSING	TEN TO TPM(200)
VARIABLES	EN1, TIRED ALL THE TIME/
	P1, PAIN AT NIGHT/
	EM1, THINGS ARE GETTING HIM DOWN/
	P2, UNBEARABLE PAIN/
	SL1, NEEDS TABLETS TO SLEEP/
	EM2, HAS FORGOTTEN HOW TO ENJOY HIMSELF/
	EM3, FEELING ON EDGE/
	P3, PAINFUL TO CHANGE POSITION/
	SO1, FEELS LONELY/
	PM1, CAN ONLY WALK INDOORS/
	PM2, HARD TO BEND/
	EN2, EVERYTHING IS AN EFFORT/
	SL2, WAKES UP EARLY/
	PM3, IS UNABLE TO WALK AT ALL/
	SO2, FINDS IT HARD TO CONTACT PEOPLE/
	EM4, THE DAYS DRAG/
	PM4, FINDS STAIRS OR STEPS DIFFICULT/
	PM5, FINDS IT HARD TO REACH FOR THINGS/
	P4, HAS PAIN WHEN WALKS/
	EM5, LOSES TEMPER EASILY/
	SO3, CAN NOT GET CLOSE TO ANYONE/
	SL3, LIES AWAKE FOR MOST OF THE NIGHT/
	EM6, THINKS HE IS LOSING CONTROL/
	P5, HAS PAIN WHEN STANDING/
	PM6, FINDS IT HARD TO DRESS/

Coding of Part I Responses by Computer Programme (cont)

EN3, SOON LOSES ENERGY/
PM7, FINDS IT HARD TO STAND FOR
LONG/
P6, IS IN CONSTANT PAIN/
SL4, TAKES A LONG TIME TO GET TO
SLEEP/
SO4, FEELS HE IS A BURDEN TO OTHERS
/EM7, WORRY KEEPS HIM AWAKE/
EM8, FEELS THAT LIFE IS NOT WORTH
LIVING/
SL5, SLEEPS BADLY AT NIGHT/
SO5, FINDS IT HARD TO WALK OUTSIDE/
P7, HAS PAIN WHEN USING STAIRS OR
STEPS/
EM9, WAKES UP DEPRESSED/
P8, HAS PAIN WHEN SITTING/

ANALYSIS

For fairly large groups, say N>20, it is possible to compute the mean of the weighted scores on Part I for comparison purposes. However, for smaller numbers or for individuals, mean scores will be misleading and it is preferable to calculate the mean rank score for the small group. This is also the case if a high percentage of the sample have zero scores on all sections.

Non-parametric statistics are the best choice for analysis of the data as it is unlikely to be normally distributed. On Part I a Mann-Whitney U-test is to be preferred for the comparison of two independent groups; the Kruskal-Wallis one-way analysis of variance for comparing three or more groups; the Wilcoxon matched-pairs signed ranks test for matched groups and a Friedman two-way analysis of variance for analysing repeated measures on the same group of people.

On Part II independent groups can be compared by means of the chi-squared test. With repeated measures the McNemar test should be used in the two-sample case and the Cochran Q test for more than two repeated measures.

Part I provides a profile of perceived health problems in the areas of energy, pain, emotional reactions, sleep, social isolation and physical mobility.

Part II gives a guide to how perceived health

problems are affecting areas of daily living.

It may not always be necessary to have the information provided by Part II and it may then be omitted.

Part II is best used with specific groups eg the chronically ill or patients who suffer from the same disease, in order to see where health problems are having most impact. For group comparisons the percentage of people in each group who answer affirmatively can be calculated, but this may obscure important differences between sub-groups and individuals.

AGE AND SEX NORMS

Several studies have indicated important age and sex differences in scores. Women usually have higher scores than men and scores tend to rise with age.

Table 7 provides age and sex 'norms' for Part I and Table 8 for Part II. These have been drawn from a random sample in the community (n=2173). It must be emphasised that these norms provide only a rough guide to 'normal' scores for groups and have been obtained only from the Nottingham area.

Scores illustrating social class differences (using the Registrar General's classification) are shown in Tables 9 and 10.

Table 11 shows mean scores from various groups used in the studies previously described.

ADVANTAGES OF THE NHP

1. Suitability for use in a wide range of situations from individual clinical interviews to large scale postal surveys.
2. High reliability and validity.
3. Easy and cheap to administer.
4. Takes only a short time to complete and is highly acceptable to respondents.
5. Easy to score and compute. Particularly suited for experimental analysis using the Statistical Package for the Social Sciences.
6. Since the NHP does not ask directly if people have health problems it is more likely to pick up people who are ill or at risk but who do not perceive their problems as being related to health.
7. Scores can be compared graphically.

Table 7: Age and Sex Norms on Part I (mean scores) (General Practice sample)

		20-24	25-29	30-34	35-39	40-44	45-49
Energy	M	10.1	8.6	4.0	5.0	10.1	8.0
	F	16.6	20.0	14.7	14.1	12.6	17.0
Pain	M	0.7	1.6	2.8	2.6	5.8	3.0
	F	1.1	2.8	3.0	1.5	5.9	7.0
Emotional	M	11.6	10.3	6.3	10.3	10.4	7.7
Reactions	F	14.3	14.7	11.2	17.9	10.0	13.1
Sleep	M	8.4	8.6	6.2	5.7	11.9	8.4
	F	12.1	9.7	13.1	11.8	13.0	15.2
Social	M	5.5	5.6	2.9	2.7	5.0	1.6
Isolation	F	7.1	6.9	4.3	7.4	3.5	5.3
Physical	M	1.5	1.6	1.3	1.2	3.2	1.1
Mobility	F	1.4	2.0	1.9	1.0	3.3	4.1

Table 7 (cont): Age and Sex Norms on Part I (mean scores) (General Practice sample)

		50-54	55-59	60-64	65-69	70-74	75+
Energy	M	11.6	13.3	15.5	13.8	20.0	29.3
	F	1.8	18.6	18.7	23.6	34.3	44.0
Pain	M	7.1	2.9	8.3	8.8	7.3	14.1
	F	6.0	14.5	10.0	20.9	16.4	25.9
Emotional	M	10.6	7.7	9.9	5.3	8.7	12.8
Reactions	F	9.3	11.2	10.0	12.5	14.5	16.6
Sleep	M	13.4	11.7	19.8	19.9	16.8	30.6
	F	16.7	20.3	20.1	38.5	30.4	29.9
Social	M	5.5	3.4	7.4	2.7	4.2	9.8
Isolation	F	5.3	5.3	6.0	5.9	10.7	12.1
Physical	M	4.1	3.7	7.5	7.3	9.6	21.3
Mobility	F	4.8	7.4	8.6	18.0	16.9	36.1

Manual

Table 8: Age and Sex Norms on Part II (mean scores) (General Practice sample)

		20-24	25-29	30-34	35-39	40-44	45-49
		%	%	%	%	%	%
Work	M	3.5	7.0	4.3	12.7	13.7	5.3
	F	5.9	6.3	3.5	13.4	9.1	5.2
Looking	M	4.4	6.2	0.0	3.2	9.7	7.1
after the	F	12.6	13.2	9.4	17.9	14.1	11.2
home							
Social	M	5.3	8.6	2.9	6.3	9.7	1.8
life	F	10.1	11.3	4.7	10.4	8.4	5.9
Home life	M	7.8	8.6	2.9	4.8	9.7	8.0
	F	10.1	16.3	12.9	22.4	12.0	11.1
Sex life	M	6.1	6.2	2.9	3.2	13.7	9.8
	F	11.8	23.2	11.8	23.9	14.1	15.5
Interests	M	7.0	14.1	2.9	4.8	14.5	11.6
& hobbies	F	7.6	10.1	5.9	14.9	6.3	10.4
Holidays	M	6.1	6.2	1.4	3.2	8.1	5.3
	F	5.9	5.0	3.5	5.9	5.6	7.4

Table 8 (cont): Age and Sex Norms on Part II (mean scores) (General Practice sample)

		50-54	55-59	60-64	65-69	70-74	75+
		%	%	%	%	%	%
Work	M	26.5	13.8	19.1	1.4	4.0	0.0
	F	9.6	8.4	4.2	8.2	1.5	0.0
Looking	M	11.7	12.3	13.2	10.9	24.3	30.5
after the	F	13.7	16.9	12.7	28.8	33.0	40.8
home							
Social	M	14.7	6.1	10.3	10.1	21.6	26.7
life	F	10.9	9.8	9.8	20.5	26.1	33.8

261

Table 8 (cont): Age and Sex Norms on Part II
(mean scores) (General Practice sample)

		50-54	55-59	60-64	65-69	70-74	75+
		%	%	%	%	%	%
Home life	M	13.2	6.1	0.0	2.9	9.4	9.7
	F	5.5	2.8	4.2	6.8	10.8	11.3
Sex life	M	20.6	18.5	10.3	14.5	18.9	18.0
	F	12.3	21.7	7.0	15.1	12.7	7.0
Interests	M	14.7	10.8	20.6	11.6	24.3	26.7
& hobbies	F	10.9	7.0	11.3	19.2	22.2	22.5
Holidays	M	13.2	4.6	11.8	13.0	21.6	36.1
	F	9.6	11.3	12.7	19.2	26.1	31.0

Table 9: Mean Scores on Part I of the Profile by Social Class (Males and Females, all ages)

SOCIAL CLASS	I (n=76)	II (n=279)	IIIN (n=249)	IIIM (n=467)	IV (n=165)	V (n=61)
ENERGY	10.25	10.63	15.69	15.84	18.58	13.49
PAIN	3.00	4.70	6.84	7.60	6.51	8.24
EMOTIONAL REACTIONS	9.74	8.42	9.00	9.89	14.41	13.07
SLEEP	7.60	9.86	14.83	15.95	20.89	22.29
SOCIAL ISOLATION	4.98	3.78	4.50	4.27	7.51	5.45
PHYSICAL MOBILITY	3.05	3.12	5.58	6.42	5.20	7.66

Table 10: Percentage of Affirmative Responses on Areas of Daily Life being affected by Health problems by Social Class (Males and Females, all ages) (Part II of the Profile)

SOCIAL CLASS	I (n=76)	II (n=279)	IIIN (n=249)	IIIM (n=467)	IV (n=165)	V (n=6)
PAID EMPLOYMENT	5.2	6.1	8.09	8.1	9.7	21.3
JOBS AROUND THE HOUSE	6.5	9.6	15.3	13.5	15.1	9.8
SOCIAL LIFE	5.2	6.4	12.8	11.3	12.1	16.3
PERSONAL RELATIONSHIPS	7.9	5.0	7.2	8.8	11.5	6.5
SEX LIFE	10.5	12.2	13.6	13.7	12.1	8.1
HOBBIES & INTERESTS	10.5	7.2	14.4	13.3	15.1	16.3
HOLIDAYS	6.2	3.9	11.2	11.1	14.5	6.5

Table 11: Mean Scores on Sections of Part I for Selected Groups

	Mine Rescue Workers	'Fit' Elderly	Pregnancy 18 wks	Pregnancy 37 wks	Patients with minor non-acute conditions
ENERGY	0.99	4.06	31.4	39.6	24.2
PAIN	1.37	1.05	2.1	11.2	15.9
EMOTIONAL REACTIONS	1.25	3.28	15.7	15.7	14.7
SLEEP	4.21	0.68	11.3	28.3	18.7
SOCIAL ISOLATION	0.38	1.34	6.4	6.2	5.1
PHYSICAL MOBILITY	0.54	1.91	7.3	26.0	7.3

Table 11 (cont): Mean Scores on Sections of Part I for Selected Groups

	Fracture victims	Patients with Peripheral Vascular Disease	Chronically ill elderly	Patients with osteo-arthrosis
ENERGY	25.79	30.3	37.98	63.2
PAIN	26.58	22.6	29.16	70.8
EMOTIONAL REACTIONS	13.65	13.9	15.13	21.3
SLEEP	27.96	24.7	32.09	48.7
SOCIAL ISOLATION	7.99	9.2	12.80	12.5
PHYSICAL MOBILITY	27.62	22.0	29.16	54.8

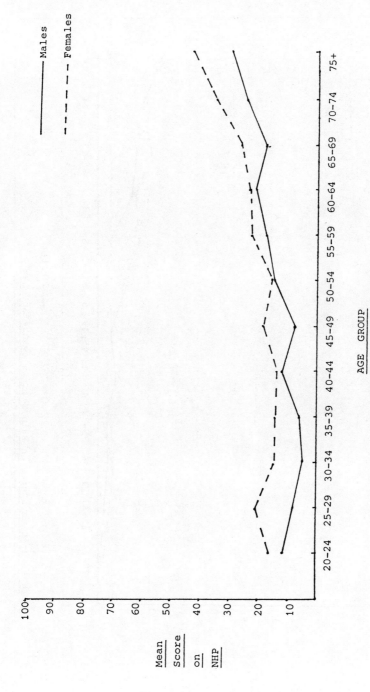

Figure 1: Mean scores on Energy section by age and sex

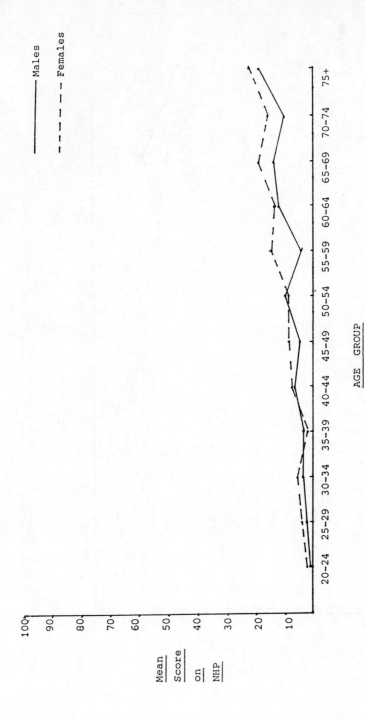

Figure 2: Mean scores on Pain section by age and sex

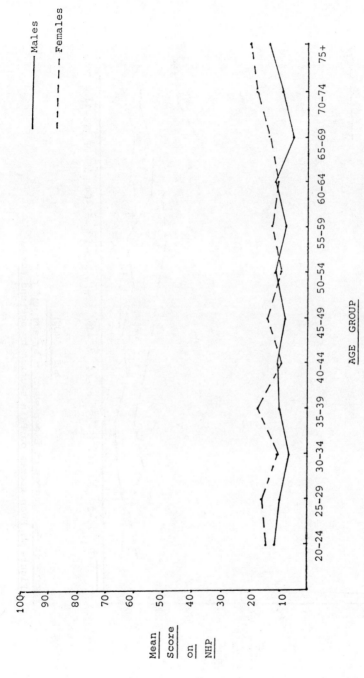

Figure 3: Mean scores on Emotional Reactions section by age and sex

269

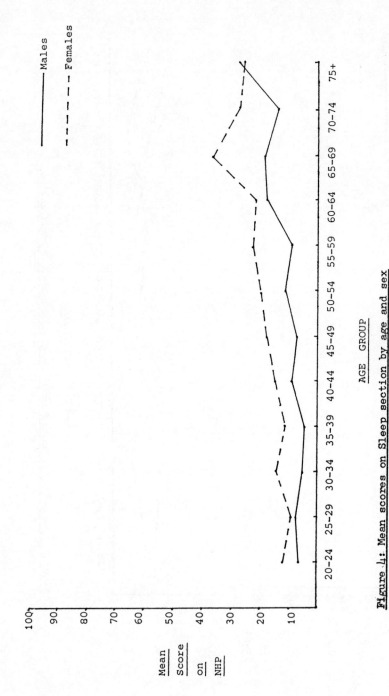

Figure 4: Mean scores on Sleep section by age and sex

270

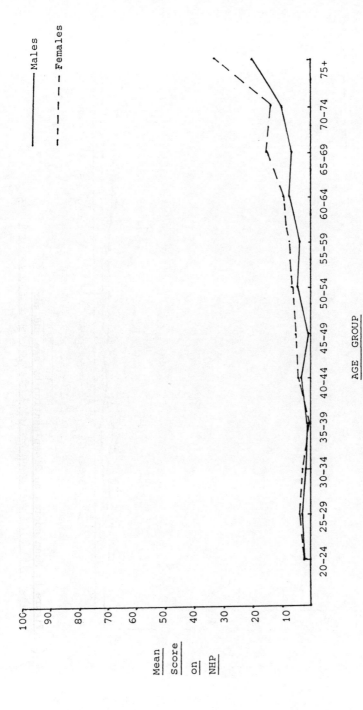

Figure 5: Mean scores on Physical Mobility section by age and sex

271

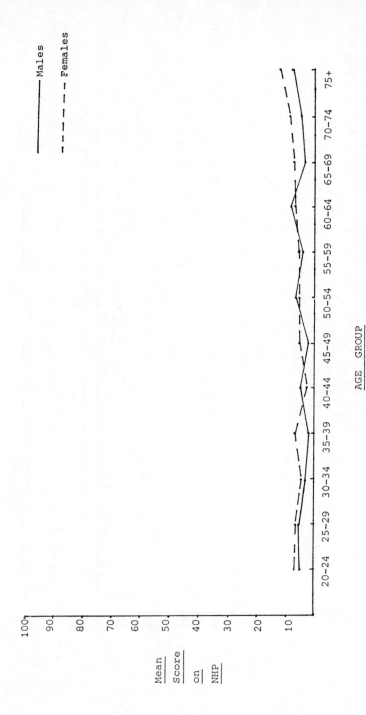

Figure 6: Mean scores on Social Isolation section by age and sex

272

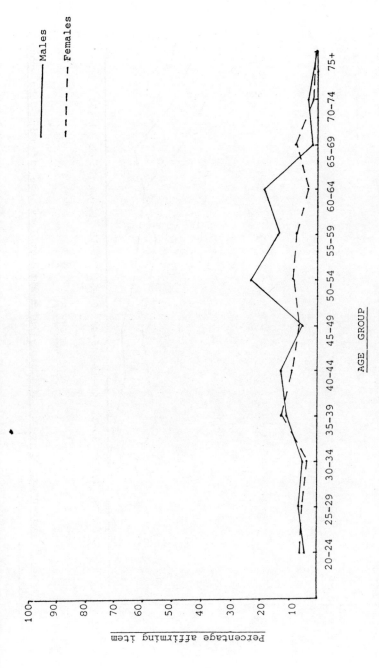

Figure 7: Percentage of people affirming that health problems were affecting Job of Work

273

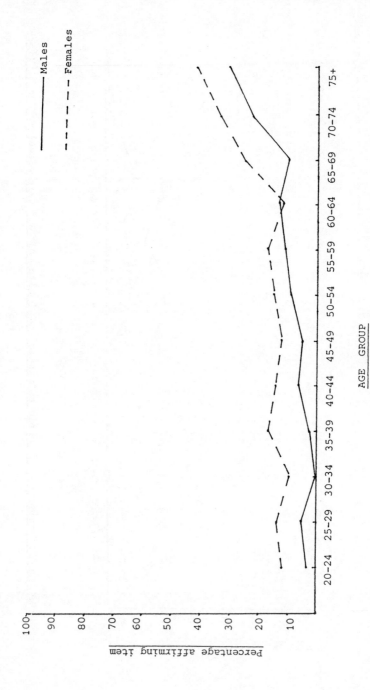

Figure 8: Percentage of people affirming that health problems were affecting Jobs around the House

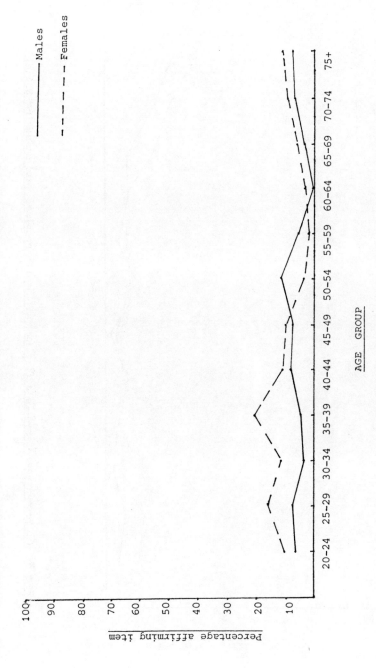

Figure 9: Percentage of people affirming that health problems were affecting Home Life

275

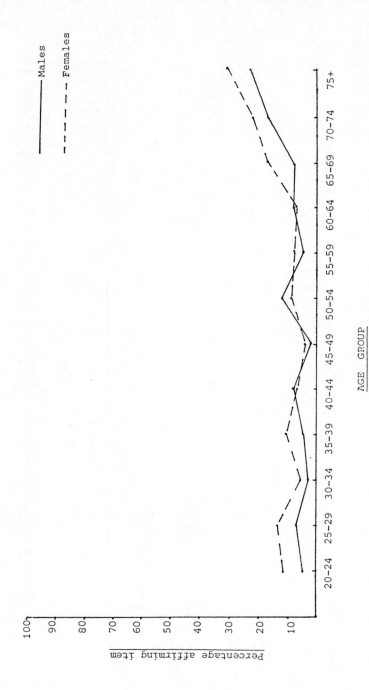

Figure 10: Percentage of people affirming that health problems were affecting Social Life

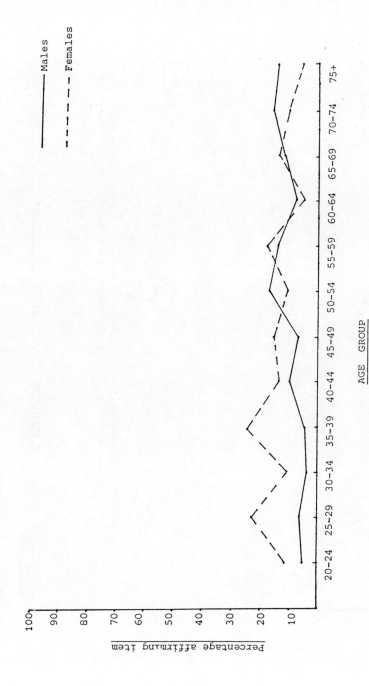

Figure 11: Percentage of people affirming that health problems were affecting Sex Life

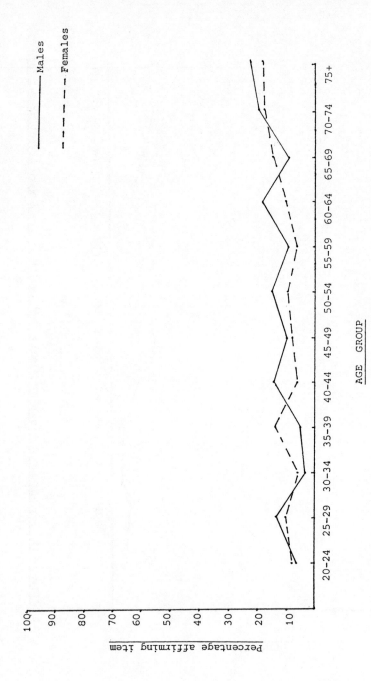

Figure 12: Percentage of people affirming that health problems were affecting Interests and Hobbies

278

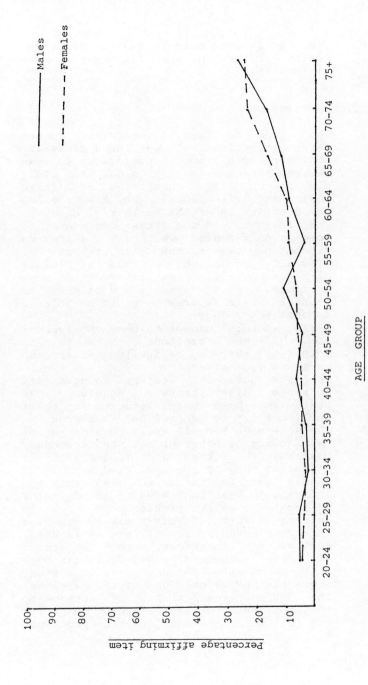

Figure 13: Percentage of people affirming that health problems were affecting Holidays

8. Can be used to measure general perceived health status and specific conditions of ill-health.

LIMITATIONS OF THE NHP

1. The items on Part I represent rather severe situations. It was found necessary to have such items in preference to less severe statements in order to avoid picking up large quantities of 'false positives' ie people who are feeling temporarily 'under the weather'. However, the severity of the items does mean that some individuals who are suffering discomfort may not show up on the NHP.

2. 'Normal' populations or those with minor ailments may affirm few statements on some sections. This makes it difficult to compare their scores, or to be able to demonstrate change.

3. 'Zero scorers' cannot be shown to improve on the NHP sections, although in actuality they may be feeling better than on a previous occasion.

4. The NHP does not attempt to cover all possible disabilities. However, the statements have been selected for their applicability to general health status.

5. The scores on Part II are a combination of two factors: whether or not the respondent has a health problem, and, if so, if it is affecting any of the specified areas. It should not be taken to mean that the individual has that area affected in the absence of a health problem.

6. Scoring on Part I involves six scores plus a further seven scores if Part II is used. Analysis can, therefore, become cumbersome if large numbers of other variables need to be taken into account, e.g. in a study where the NHP is only one of the measures.

7. The NHP measures health by its absence by focusing on negative aspects of health i.e. all the statements describe problems.

Manual

ACKNOWLEDGEMENTS

We gratefully acknowledge the help, support, advice
and contributions of the following people:

    Citizens   of   Nottingham   and   surrounding
counties;   patients   attending   clinics   at   the
Universty,   City,   General   and   Women's   Hospitals
Nottingham   and   their   relatives   and   friends.
Professor W. Waugh and consultants in the Department
of Orthopaedic Surgery; Mr B. Hopkinson of the
Department of Surgery; Professor P. Fentem, Dr E.J.
Bassey and staff of the Department of Physiology and
Pharmacology; General Practice part-time lecturers,
especially Drs P. Baldwin, A. Murphy, J. Skinner
and N. McCoach, of the Department of Community
Health, Queen's Medical Centre, Nottingham. The
nursing and auxiliary staff of the out-patient
clinics of Surgery and Orthopaedic Surgery, General
Hospital and Fracture clinic, ENT, library, catering
and portering staff of the Queen's Medical Centre.
Mrs Abbot, Mansfield Day Centre. Staff of the
Department   of   Obstetrics   and   Gynaecology,   City
Hospital, Nottingham; staff and clients of the
Family Planning Clinic, Regent Street, Nottingham.
Ms Freda Fitton and colleagues of the Department of
General   Practice,   University   Medical   School,
University   of   Manchester.   Mr   Maurice   Vaughan,
Rochester   Medical   School,   New   York.   Mr   Peter
Beynon, Adult Literacy Scheme, Nottingham. The
National   Coal   Board;   the   Boots   Co   Ltd,   the
Nottinghamshire Fire Service. Dr J. Pearson, Mr I.
Turner,   Dr Jan Davison, Dr A. Rector, Mr P.
Clements, Mrs A. Zomorski and Mr G. Widdowson,
Department   of   Community   Health,   Queen's   Medical
Centre, Nottingham.

The Social Science Research Council for their Grants
No's HR3607 and HR6157/1.

LIST OF PEOPLE ON THE RESEARCH TEAM

1975-1978   E. Backett
              J. Boyd
              J. Lindsay
              C.J.M. Martini
              I. McDowell
              E. Papp
              J. Williams

Manual

1978-1982   E. Backett
              P. Barnes
              J. Boyd
              S. Dhalakia
              L. Hart
              S. Hunt
              J. Lindsay
              J. McEwen
              S.P. McKenna
              E. Papp
              C. Pope
              J. Reeve
              D. Turner
              K. Waters
              J. Williams

REFERENCES

Backett, E.M. McEwen, J. Hunt, S.M. (1981) Report to
    the Social Science Research Council. Health
    and Quality of Life
Hunt, S.M. McKenna, S.P. McEwen, J. Backett, E.M.
    Williams, J. and Papp, E. (1980) 'A
    Quantitative Approach to Perceived Health
    Status: A Validation Study', J Epidem Comm
    Hlth, 34, 281-286
Hunt, S.M. McKenna, S.P. McEwen, J. Williams, J. and
    Papp, E. (1981) 'The Nottingham Health Profile:
    Subjective Health Status and Medical
    Consultations', Soc Sci Med, 15A, 221-229
Hunt, S.M. McKenna, S.P. Williams, J. (1981)
    'Reliabiity of a Population Survey Tool for
    measuring Perceived Health Problems: A Study of
    Patients with Osteoarthrosis', J Epid Comm
    Hlth, 35, 297-300
Hunt, S.M. McEwen, J. McKenna, S.P. Backett, E.M.
    and Pope, E. (1982) 'Subjective Health of
    Patients with Peripheral Vascular Disease', The
    Practitioner, 226, 133-136
Hunt, S.M. McEwen, J. McKenna, S.P. and Pope, C.
    (1984) 'Subjective Health Assessments and the
    Perceived Outcome of Minor Surgery', Psychosom
    Res, 28, 105-114
Hunt, S.M. McEwen, J. McKenna, S.P. (1985) 'Social
    Inequalities and Perceived Health', Effective
    Health Care, 2, 151-160
Martini, C.J.M. and McDowell, I. (1976) 'Health
    Status: Patient and Physician Judgements', Hlth
    Serv Res, Winter
Martini, C.J.M. and McDowell, I. (1977) 'The

Evaluation of Strategies for the Improvement of Life Style: An Example drawn from Two Locomotor Disorders', Paper read at a conference of the International Epidemiological Association, Puerto Rico, September

McDowell, I. Martini, C.J.M. (1976) 'Problems and New Directions in the Evaluation of Primary Care', Int J Epidem, 5, 247-50

McDowell, I. Martini, C.J.M. and Waugh, W. (1978) 'A Method for Self-Assessment of Disability before and after Hip Replacement Operations', BMJ, 2, 231-46

McEwen, J. Lowe, D. Hunt, S.M. McKenna, S.P. (1985) 'The Workplace: An Opportunity to promote Health based on the Measurement of Perceived Health', (Unpublished)

McKenna, S.P. Hunt, S.M. McEwen, J. Williams, J. and Papp, E. (1980) 'Looking at Health from the Consumer's Point of View', Occup Med, 32, 350-355

McKenna, S.P. Hunt, S.M. McEwen, J. (1981) 'Absence from Work and Perceived Health among Mine Rescue Workers', Occup Med, 31, 151-157

McKenna, S.P. Hunt, S.M. McEwen, J. (1981) 'Weighting the Seriousness of Perceived Health Problems using Thurstone's Method of Paired Comparisons', Int J Epid, 10, 93-97

McKenna, S.P. McEwen, J. Hunt, S.M. and Papp, E. (1984) 'Changes in the Perceived Health of Patients recovering from Fractures', Public Health, 98, 97-102

INDEX

absence from work 100,
   105-7
accuracy of responses
   153-4
ACORN 30-31
Activities of Daily
   Living Index 42
Arthritis Impact
   Measurement Scales
   43

Beck Depression
   Inventory 83
Black report 19, 227

cancer 195-6, 198
chemotherapy 2, 3, 4
Chinese 208-9
choice of treatment 164
community care 24, 31
Community medicine 23
Comprehensive Assess-
   ment and Referral
   Evaluation Scales 46
clinical trials 47-8,
   54, 166, 181-2, 198
compliance 165
conceptual equivalence
   211-4
consultation rate 100
Consulters 98, 124
Cornell Medical Index
   45, 99, 212

cross cultural adapt-
   ations 48, 210-5
   comparisons 203-4,
      207, 236
   equivalency of items
      217-9
cultural beliefs 207-10
   216
   bias 50

disability 37-8, 40, 44,
   51-2, 86, 163, 221,
   230, 232
   indices 40, 42-44,
      50, 210
Disease 37, 41, 49, 54,
   63-4, 148, 163, 207
   chronic 3, 21, 26,
      39, 42, 48, 54,
      97, 128, 135, 199
   see also disability,
   illness, health
   status, morbidity
Doctors 6, 8, 64-5, 81,
   100, 163, 165 see
   also general
   practitioners, health
   professionals,
   medical profession
dualism 61
DUKE - UNC Health
   Profile 46

Index

Elderly 45, 55, 68-69,
  97, 103, 118, 235
  assessment of 46,
    198
  population size 3
  elective surgery 168-
    174
Ethical Considerations
  227-229
evaluation 40, 42, 44,
  47, 54, 63, 65 67-8,
  148, 182, 228, 232,
  234

firemen 103, 124
fractures 109-113
Functional Assessment
  Inventory 45
Functional Limitation
  Profile 48

General Health
  Questionnaire 51,
  84-5, 142-3, 230
general practitioners
  26, 34, 38, 66, 98-9
  see also doctors,
  health profession-
  als, medical prof-
  ession
global index 38, 52
Griffiths report 27

handicap 42, 86, 210
Health 4, 6, 8, 37, 41,
  49, 52, 63-4, 67,
  97, 101, 109, 139,
  148, 154, 172, 230
  care 5, 19, 21, 27,
    31-4, 65, 86,
    199
  concepts 5, 37, 70,
    207, 231
  indicators 22, 33-4,
    49, 61, 203, 221,
    225-6
  choice of 54-55
  needs 5, 27, 53,
    203-4, 225
  policy 33, 52, 203-
    4, 226, 233

services 4, 7-10, 19-
  31, 33, 39, 66-7,
  99, 102, 135, 199,
  206, 226-7, 230-3
status 6, 22, 30-1,
  34, 37-8, 40-1,
  44, 46, 50-2, 63-
  8, 86, 98, 100,
  103, 114, 132,
  155, 173, 183,
  191, 203, 225, 232
surveys 34, 41-3, 48,
  54, 206, 233
Health Assessment
  Questionnaire 43
Health Belief Model 66-7
Health Goals Model 53
Health Perceptions
  Questionnaire 47
health professionals 4,
  30, 181; see also
  doctors, general
  practitioners,
  medical profession
health related behaviour
  67
Heart transplantation
  182-194, 228
Herzlich 5
Hip replacement 3, 115,
  134, 227

Illich 10, 233
Illness 5-6, 38, 51, 53,
  54, 64, 75, 86, 104,
  114, 141, 207, 230;
  see also disease,
  disability, health
  status, morbidity
impairment 42, 45, 210;
  see also disability,
  handicap
Index of Health 52
Index of Psychological
  Well-Being 49
inner city 124, 134-7,
  233; see also social
  class, social depriv-
  ation, social
  inequalities
interviewer effects 136-

7, 149
item selection 76-7,
  86-7, 107

Korner committee 26
  report 31

Langer's Mental Health
  Scale 49
linguistic relativity
  216

McMaster Health Index
  Questionnaire 46,
  117
medicalisation 233
medical profession 10,
  19, 62, 164; see
  also doctors,
  general
  practitioners,
  health professionals
mental health 45, 49,
  64
mine rescue workers
  104-5
Morbidity 19-20, 38,
  40-2, 52, 68, 99,
  111, 133-7, 141,
  144-5, 154-5, 204,
  206-10, 232; see
  also disability,
  illness, health
  status
Mortality rates 19-20,
  38-40, 52, 68, 75,
  128, 141, 145, 169,
  204-5, 230
  risk 47

National Health Service
  23, 29, 31, 66, 103
non-parametric tests
  100, 157-8
non-response 150-3
norms 55, 63, 124-48,
  235
Nottinham Health
  Profile 51, 70, 85-
  119, 124-48, 154-60,
  163-80, 183-200,

226, 229, 230-1,
  231-8
age differences
  101-2, 118, 126-
  133, 137-9, 196,
  Appendix
Arabic version 213-6
distribution of
  scores 154-7, 220,
  Appendix
limitations 235-6,
  Appendix
North american
  version 219-20
sex differences 101-
  2, 118, 126-133,
  137-9, 196,
  Appendix
Spanish version 218-9
social class
  differences 126-
  133, 137-9

objectivity 62, 67, 75,
  99
Older American's
  Resources and
  Services Inventory 45
osteoarthrosis 115, 124,
  134

parametric techniques
  157-8
perceived health 67, 68-
  70, 75-119, 124-148,
  152, 154-60, 163,
  166, 169-74, 180,
  192, 198, 219
population structure 3
positive health 43, 49,
  230-1
pregnancy 174-181
Psychological General
  Well-Being Index 49
Public health 2, 7, 10,
  21, 23

Q index 52
Quality-adjusted life
  years 53
quality of life 5, 47,

53, 66, 85, 163,
165, 182
in cancer 195
in heart transplant-
ation 194
Quality of Well-Being
Scale 47

reliability 47-51, 55,
70, 86, 92, 113-7,
139, 194, 204-5,
219, 221, 229
renal transplantation 3
reproducibility 82
resource allocation 25,
38, 39, 52-3, 87,
169, 227, 234
Resource Allocation
Working Party 45

Safwa 208
sample size 79, 149-53
Sapir-Whorf hypothesis
213
Saudia Arabia 209
scaling methods 75-85,
88-95
Guttman technique
82-3, 88
Likert method 84-5,
88
paired comparisons
77-8, 80, 81, 88-
95
rank ordering 77-8,
80, 88
rating techniques
77, 79, 80-3
scientific method 62
screening 64, 198
Self assessment 5, 45-
8, 55, 63, 68-70,
99, 101, 135, 154,
211, 213
self care 8-9, 46
semantic differential
79
semantic equivalence
211-5 see also
conceptual equiv-
alence, translation

Sepik 207-8
Sickness Impact Profile
48, 50, 117
small area analysis 227
see also ACORN
social acceptability 154
social class 31, 81, 96,
126, 141-3
social deprivation 25,
30-1, 135, 227, 233
see also social
deprivation
social reality 207
Subanun 209
subjective health 51,
67-70, 86, 95-6, 98,
101, 166, 195
factors in utilis-
ation of services
66-67
judgements of 67
measures of 40, 226
needs 86

Thurstone 78, 81-2, 84
Thyroid disease 166-8
Translation 211-3, 217
of NHP into Arabic
213-6
of NHP into Spanish
218-9
of NHP into north
american 219-20
of SIP into Spanish
217-8
see also conceptual
equivalence, semantic
equivalence

unemployment 134, 139-48
utilisation 41, 49, 51,
68, 98-9, 134

validity 44-51, 55, 70,
86, 95-107, 109, 194,
210, 218-9, 221, 229
vietnamese 212

weighting 78-81, 87-95,
108-9, 129-30, 151,
217, 220

well-being 37, 38, 43,
    64, 172, 230-1, 233
    see also quality of
        life, positive
        health
Whorf 216
World Health
    Organisation 33,
    203, 220-1, 225
    definition of health
        230